complete
colon
cleanse

D0556919

complete

the

at-home

detox

program

to

colon

cleanse

restore

DR. EDWARD F. GROUP III

good

health,

boost

vitality

and

ensure

longevity

Ulysses
Press

Text Copyright © 2007 Dr. Edward F. Group III. Design Copyright © 2007 Ulysses Press and its licensors. All rights reserved under International and Pan-American Copyright Conventions, including the right to reproduce this book or portions thereof in any form whatsoever, except for use by a reviewer in connection with a review.

Published by:
ULYSSES PRESS
P.O. Box 3440
Berkeley, CA 94703
www.ulyssespress.com

ISBN10: 1-56975-594-9
ISBN13: 978-1-56975-594-5
Library of Congress Control Number: 2007905320

Printed in the United States by Bang Printing

10 9 8 7 6 5 4 3 2 1

Acquisitions Editor: Nicholas Denton-Brown
Managing Editor: Claire Chun
Editor: Mark Woodworth
Editorial and production staff: Elyce Petker, Judith Metzener, Steven Zah Schwartz
Index: Sayre Van Young
Cover design: Double R Resign
Cover photo: ©photos.com
Interior design and layout: what!design @ whatweb.com
Interior illustrations and photos: Nida Ali

Distributed by Publishers Group West

NOTE TO READERS
This book has been written and published strictly for informational and educational purposes only. It is not intended to serve as medical advice or to be any form of medical treatment. You should always consult your physician before altering or changing any aspect of your medical treatment and/or undertaking a diet regimen, including the colon cleanse as described in this book. Do not stop or change any prescription medications without the guidance and advice of your physician. Any use of the information in this book is made on the reader's good judgment after consulting with his or her physician and is the reader's sole responsibility. This book is not intended to diagnose or treat any medical condition and is not a substitute for a physician.

This book is dedicated to *you*.

The inspiration behind my years of research has come from knowing that I'm helping people every day. You are my motivation and my passion. If it weren't for you, this book would never have been written.

So, from the bottom of my heart, thank you.

Contents

Acknowledgments

So many people in my life have supported me, believed in me, given me hope, and shared information that has literally changed my life. The list of those who deserve thanks is extremely long, but, unfortunately, my space is limited. So I'd like to extend my sincere thanks to everyone who continues to be a part of my life. I greatly appreciate the faith and support you've given me over the years.

A special thanks to my immediate family—my mother and father in the heavens above, my lovely wife Dr. Daniela Group, our newborn organic son Edward the IV, Dr. Thetis Group, Dr. Joan Roberts, Jon Group and family, Mika (Volim Te Puno), Tea and Jon Pollock, and my favorite nephew Luka. Thank you so much for all your love and support.

And, of course, thanks to the entire Global Healing Center Family—for your commitment to excellence, for all your ideas and effort day in and day out, and for believing and supporting my vision of helping people recapture their health every day.

Introduction
The Secret to Health

I'll let you in on a little secret—actually, a gigantic one. Do you want to know the single biggest reason why hundreds of millions of people around the globe suffer from poor health? The secret is that they need to regularly cleanse their body, starting with the intestines and colon, and then should take steps to reduce the toxins they ingest and absorb every day through food, water, drugs, stress, and elements in their personal environment. The good news for *you* is that this book will help you to start taking responsibility for your own health by doing internal cleansing. Unraveling this secret is my gift to you.

I've dedicated my professional life as a natural health care practitioner to finding the one thing that anyone can do to achieve better health. I firmly believe I've finally found the answer. If you wish to recover from illness, or prevent it, you need to start detoxifying your body *now*, starting with the colon. This book will tell you everything you need to know to reach optimal health. It's your step-by-step guide to securing a long-term solution. After all, what's the point of learning how to cleanse your colon if you're just going to fall back into the same disease-causing habits? While it's easy for me to tell you all the ways you can tackle the symptoms of disease, in fact the real answers come when you yourself learn how to address the root causes of problems affecting your health—and then follow through.

So now let me tell you my secrets to overcoming disease and living a happier, healthier life.

I am truly excited to share with you my conclusions from years of research, just as I recently did at the International Science and Consciousness Conference in Santa Fe, New Mexico. Addressing a large gathering of international scientists, natural health care practitioners, and medical doctors, I revealed one of the most overlooked and suppressed health secrets in the world. I told them how we all should regard it as tragic that this information has been withheld from the general public and not been included as a part of standard medical training. After 15 years of research I have finally pieced everything together. I am positive this information is the key to preventing disease and healing the body naturally.

For years, I have focused on helping my patients understand and practice good, regular internal body cleansing. I have worked with them intensively and have witnessed the prevention or outright disappearance of practically every disease known to medicine. I often tell my clients that looking to science for answers is often unproductive or even damaging, when in fact the explanation is usually quite simple and staring them in the face.

I want to share this groundbreaking information with you, as well—because I know that you want to maximize your health and perhaps even help your friends and family regain their own well-being and prevent disease down the road.

As this book explains in detail, the intestines are the first point of attack for the majority of all disease-causing agents. Toxins and parasites make their way by the millions every day into the bloodstream via the intestinal tract, subsequently causing toxic blood, thereby overworking the liver and infiltrating every type of tissue. This process, I believe, is the origin of the "dis-ease" mechanism. A small amount of harmful toxins enter through the skin and lungs via direct contact and respiration. The disease-causing agents include internal parasites, as well as massive amounts of toxins from food, water, stress, drugs, and other things.

When the intestines become toxic, they can't properly absorb nutrients from food, because they are packed with layers of old, impacted waste material. This creates a narrowed passageway, leading to constipation and other bowel problems. If toxins are not regularly eliminated from the intestines, they leach back into the bloodstream through what is termed "leaky gut syndrome" and ultimately cause disease.

But why, you ask, is this role of the intestines such a big secret? Maybe "lack of knowledge" is a better term. Ask any doctor to explain the role of the intestines in detail and how they function in the body, and I guarantee that they will not be able to give you a definitive answer.

Medical science can explain the function of every organ in the body except the appendix. Sound strange? Well, why do you think so many people have their appendix removed (more than 200,000 appendectomies are done each year in the United States)? Doctors still don't know what the appendix is, much less what it does. Standard treatment methods as taught in medical schools dictate removing that organ whenever it becomes inflamed. Why? The medical industry realizes a simple truth—without your appendix, you are destined for disease, so doctors can sell you more drugs, perform more unnecessary surgeries, or (even worse) treat you with deadly radiation as a "cure" that's definitely worse than the disease. But why is the appendix so important? Here's my theory: It's located at the juncture of the small and large intestines, where it acts as a body regulator and communicator. It monitors internal pH, the toxic load present, and the opening and closing of the ileocecal valve, plus it sends messages to the immune system regarding activity in the bowel. The appendix is made up of lymphoid tissue (immune cells) and it regulates lymphatic, exocrine, endocrine, and neuromuscular functions. The appendix acts as a microcomputer relay station for the body. You might be wondering— why would the body's regulatory computer be located in the colon, of all places? My answer is—why *wouldn't* it be?

Why are doctors not taught to prevent disease, instead of addressing the symptoms of disease? After all, if preventive measures and cleansing were taught in medical schools, many diseases we take for granted would simply cease to exist. The gargantuan pharmaceutical industry, those massively government-funded medical research studies, and those entire armies of around-the-clock medical staff in every city and town across the land would mostly be unnecessary if people discovered that all they had to do to achieve optimal health was to keep their intestines, liver, and body clean. (Might we then find better uses for the hundreds of billions of dollars our country spends on so-called "health care"?)

Maybe doctors, just like ordinary folks, are embarrassed to talk about bodily eliminations of waste, thinking them taboo topics. All too often, the digestive system and the colon in particular have the status of being "second-class organs" because we view them as being too nasty or dirty to discuss. Yet, consider for a moment how important these components are in the grand scheme of biological living. The intestines are the first exposure point to, and thus the first line of defense against, a host of toxins to which we expose ourselves every day. After years of toxic buildup, the liver (another vital organ) also takes a beating and must be cleansed regularly.

When I had my natural health practice, I took on the hardest cancer and degenerative disease cases I could find—because I loved the challenge. Patients would sometimes ask me during the initial consultation, "What are you going to do for me that all the other doctors couldn't do?" I would reply, "Let me ask *you* a question: What did all the other doctors do to cleanse or detoxify your body *before* giving you bottles of prescription drugs or bags of supplements?" Practically every one of them would respond with confusion, "Cleanse? What's that?"

Well, I didn't just tell them. I *showed* my patients the positive effects that cleansing could have on their health and explained to them that their body is the best doctor they have. I told them that when their bodies are clean they activate their own self-healing mechanism. Coming back to see me, they would often report in amazement that half their symptoms had already disappeared, even though I hadn't even begun to treat their condition. Their results came solely from the cleansing regimen I devised for them. I would then assure them, in all modesty, that I don't actually "heal" anyone, for true healing comes from within; it's every person's responsibility to heal himself or herself. The definition of a true doctor is: *A teacher, not a prescriber*. Teaching someone like you how to heal is my responsibility—indeed, it's my moral obligation—as a true doctor.

This book, then, is designed to teach you how to heal yourself and activate your own self-healing mechanism. In Part 1, I share with you my "Secret to Health"—eliminating as many toxins as you can, regularly (or even daily), before they reach and infect your intestines and go on to cause disease. Then, in Part 2, I tell you the ways you absorb or are exposed to toxins, through food and drink, air and water, medications and stress, heavy metals and radiation, and parasites. Throughout the book, I offer many practical, specific ways in which you can reduce or eliminate toxins, conquer your unhealthy food addictions, and deal firmly with toxin-delivering mechanisms you may never have even known about. Along the way, I list techniques you can use to reprogram some of your "bad" habits. In the back of the book, I include a section on wide-ranging resources for products and services to assist you, as well as a glossary of important terms and medical conditions.

Once people start cleansing internally to regain their health, emotional disorders often go away. Do you ever go about your day feeling as if you're in a fog, like everything is slightly out of focus or you can't concentrate the way you used to? This perpetual haze isn't caused by the natural aging process alone. Your mental clarity is affected by the toxic substances you consume. The toxic chemicals disrupt our sensitive biochemical and hormonal regulation by altering the electrical signals in the water surrounding our cells and in our blood. The resulting disruption in the brain and liver causes depression, mood disorders, and other emotional disturbances

Think about the last time you felt really healthy. Take a moment to remember how your mind and body and spirit felt. You probably were self-confident and eager to face the day, because you looked and felt *great*. You actually loved yourself and desired to experience life in its rich variety. You enjoyed your connections with other people in your life, your community, the larger world. Well, I assure you that if you take to heart and practice the "secret" that I detail in this book, you can feel that way again. When you cleanse your body regularly, and deal with bad health habits generally, you can regain your self-confidence and sense of self and even hope for the future. You can again believe that you are capable of achieving anything you put your mind to. This encourages success in anything you manifest through your thoughts and actions.

No more secrets. I wish you happiness and well-being—and I wish you better colon health!

PART I

Health Begins in the Colon

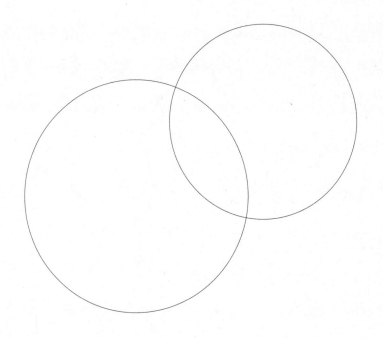

CHAPTER 1

What Is a Toxic Colon?

If you have not read "Secret to Health" in the Introduction, please go back and read it now. It will give you a much better understanding of everything I have written in this book.

Let's pretend for a moment that your body is a car. Every 3,000 miles or so, you need to have your oil and filters changed because they've become caked with sticky, black grunge from your engine. This buildup of polluted sludge forces your engine to work harder and harder to keep the tires rolling. All this extra work increases the wear and tear on the engine, and if something isn't done about it, sooner or later it's going to break down.

But most of us drive our cars for only a few hours each day, and have our oil changed once every two or three months. Your body, by contrast, runs 24 hours a day, 7 days a week, 365 days a year. And most of us go years and years without cleaning the inside of our bodies.

In a lot of ways, your colon is like the exhaust pipe that runs underneath your car. The gas in your fuel tank is sucked into the engine where it's mixed with air and oil to create the fire that moves the pistons that create the energy that ultimately makes the wheels turn, and finally the exhaust fumes are expelled. This is a complicated process that requires a near-perfect balance of various mechanical, electrical, and chemical reactions. And, as with any reaction, these processes create certain byproducts or toxins. In the case of your car, those toxins are exhaust emissions.

Your body works in much the same way. The foods you eat are pumped from your stomach into your intestines where they are combined and broken down to create the energy that ultimately keeps you moving. The foods you fuel your body with also create certain byproducts. If the intestines are functioning properly, these byproducts are expelled two to four times a day through regular bowel movements.

Do you know what happens when your car's engine isn't running smoothly and its exhaust pipe gets congested with polluted gunk? It backfires. So what do you think happens to your body when your colon gets congested with *its* own kind of gunk?

Have you ever seen a rusted-out exhaust pipe with holes in it? Besides making it difficult to pass an emissions test, these holes can allow toxic exhaust fumes to leak into the cab of your car.

With time, your colon can also develop holes, which allow toxins to leak into your bloodstream. Eventually these toxins find their way into other organs and bodily tissues where they fester and cause disease.

Over the last 100 years or so, humankind has polluted the air, the food, the water, and practically everything else we've been able to get our hands on. Many of us just stand around watching all these developments go on around us, and think, "Well, nothing will really affect me." Or we go to a documentary movie about global warming, or listen to a story on the news about a new and alarming source of pollution, and think we're not involved.

Think again. Our bodies *are* absorbing this toxic pollution. And the harsh reality is that one in every two people is developing some form of cancer. Today we are faced with more disease than ever before.

It may seem hard to believe, but basically all the toxins that I will talk about in this book (and that's a *lot* of them) enter the body through our mouth, our nose, or our skin, and are absorbed directly through our intestines.

Most people think that the toxins they consume affect only their liver and kidneys, but that isn't the whole truth. Even though these organs process as many toxins as they possibly can, in about 8 out of 10 people over the age of 30 the liver becomes overwhelmed and the overall toxin load in the body rises to above normal. They eventually have no choice but to dump the excess back into the body.

Normally, the liver tries to convert substances it receives from the digestive system into nutrients we can use. The problem is, both our liver and our intestines are faced with more toxins than they can possibly handle. They quickly get caught in a vicious cycle of passing toxins back and forth. All our organs are dangerously overworked—especially our intestines.

Before going any further, I'd like to make something clear. For ease of reading, I will be referring to the "colon" and the "intestines" as one entity. While this is a book about colon cleansing, simply focusing on the colon without concentrating on the full intestinal tract would be addressing only half the problem. The small intestine *and* the colon (or large intestine) must *both* be cleansed regularly to achieve better health.

Another word you're going to see used a lot in this book is "toxin." By strict definition, a toxin is a substance of organic origin that is damaging to living tissue. But again, for the sake of simplicity, I'll be using "toxin" generically to mean any foreign substance that wreaks havoc on your health once it's inside your body. Because in the end, whether we're talking about airborne pollutants from a refinery or the toxic byproduct of yeast overgrowth in your intestines, the results are the same—disease and a toxic colon.

Although some general understanding of the inner workings of the colon and its processes will greatly enhance your experience as you read this book, they are by no means necessary. And so, without further ado, let's do a quick and painless overview of the anatomy and physiology of the colon.

What Exactly Does the Colon Do?

The colon, or large intestine, is one of the primary components of your digestive system. It's made up of basically the same types of tissues found in your throat, stomach, and small intestines, though the colon has a few unique characteristics that set it apart from the rest of the digestive tract. For one thing, no part of the large intestine produces digestive enzymes. That's left entirely to the small intestine. The colon itself is divided into four parts—the *ascending colon*, the *transverse colon*, the *descending colon*, and the *sigmoid colon*. To get an idea of their arrangement, see Figure 1 on page 4.

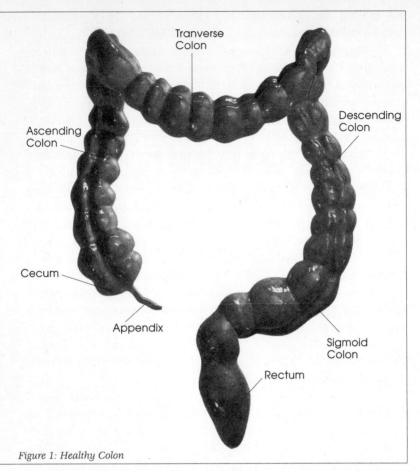

Figure 1: Healthy Colon

After leaving the small intestine, waste enters the ascending colon on the right side of the abdomen. As you might have guessed, the ascending colon moves waste upward to the transverse colon, which spans the gap to the descending colon, which in turn carries waste downward and out through the rectum.

Most of the vitamins and nutrients that our bodies pull from the foods we eat have already been absorbed by the small intestine before reaching the colon. The colon's primary job is to absorb the water that's left over, so that it can condense soft waste into solid waste. It also takes in select water-tied nutrients such as electrolytes. But, as you will soon find out, the colon and small intestine can also absorb dangerous toxins, and unfortunately these toxins are the root cause of nearly *all* degenerative disease.

A healthy colon is essential to your overall well-being. It's more than just a tube for the food you eat to pass through on its way out—in fact, it's a key part of the digestive process. When the colon stops functioning properly, digestion gets disrupted and the essential vitamins, minerals, and other nutrients your body depends on to grow and thrive may not be absorbed. Not only that, but an unhealthy colon is also less able to expel the toxins that it encounters.

What Causes the Colon to Malfunction in the First Place?

The foods we eat obviously have a lot to do with keeping our colons healthy. But if maintaining our colons were as easy as making a few small changes to our dietary habits, why does incidence of disease continue to skyrocket, even among people with seemingly healthy diets? The answer goes beyond our diets—it stems from our *constant exposure to everyday toxins*.

Day in and day out, we wade through a sea of toxic substances that our bodies simply aren't designed to handle. We eat food tainted with chemicals, and we drink contaminated water and beverages. We breathe polluted smog instead of oxygen-rich, clean air. And when we do finally notice that our bodies are beginning to break down, most of us go to a medical doctor for help.

We all know what happens next. These doctors prescribe synthetic, manufactured drugs that our bodies are not designed or equipped to handle. True, they may help to alleviate our symptoms for a while, but *they do nothing to actually treat the root cause of the disease*.

Believe it or not, nearly every disease known to medical science is caused, triggered, or amplified by a toxic colon. And, as I explained in the Introduction, nearly every toxin that enters the body does so through the intestinal tract. The problem is this—toxins don't always find their way out in a timely manner. They become trapped in intestinal mucous tissues, crippling the whole digestive system. This gives these toxins time to leak their way back into our bodies. This weakens our bodies and further slows down our intestinal processing.

Unfortunately, to date, the vast majority of members of the medical establishment fail to accept how critical maintaining a clean intestinal tract is to a person's health. Not just their digestive health, their overall health.

I Think I See a Pattern Emerging

If toxins are not eliminated regularly from the colon, they "leak" into the bloodstream through what we call leaky gut syndrome (see Figure 16 on page 104), and cause degenerative diseases throughout the body that cause affected tissues to deteriorate over time.

All right, so where exactly do all these toxins come from? And, more importantly, what can you and I do to prevent them and maintain our precious health? You already know that our environment is in pretty sad shape. But do you know the specific reasons why these things are hurting us? Or how exactly they're doing it?

The environment to which you expose yourself is what causes disease. Very few of us take proactive steps to shield our bodies from toxins, much less fight against the big businesses and industries that are responsible for creating them in the first place. To fully grasp the effects of toxins on your body, you must first understand the personal factors that are unique to your body. How healthy are the foods with which you fuel your body? Do you get enough exercise each day? And, most often overlooked, how high is your personal toxic threshold?

How Clogged Are Our Colons?

More than 40 million people in the United States are overweight. I'd say that's pretty clogged. The Center for Health and Health Care in Schools at George Washington University reports that "The percent of school-age children 6–11 that are overweight more than doubled between the late 1970s and 2000, rising from 6.5% to 15.3%. The percent of overweight adolescents ages 12–19 tripled from 5.0% to 15.5% during the same time period." These days, poor adult health can often be traced to poor habits developed during childhood.

What do these findings reveal? Sure, they tell us that we are raising obese kids to be obese adults, but if we carefully read between the lines, they also tell us that generations of Americans are spending their entire lives constipated. Yes, today's overweight children will likely grow up to be tomorrow's obese adults, according to current predictions. But we can put an end to these statistics and prevent these children from becoming obese.

But first we have to understand what that has to do with a toxic colon.

This epidemic trend toward increased body fat might not seem closely related to colon toxicity, but it does help illustrate two things that are both common causes of colon toxicity: *poor diet and lack of exercise.*

A well-balanced diet is essential to staying lean, healthy, and toxin-free. But the sudden spike on the bathroom scale may actually have less to do with what goes into your body than it does with what comes out of it—or, in this case, what doesn't. Often it's the same fatty foods that are synonymous with an increase in weight that lead to clogged colons.

Believe it or not, the hardened waste that obstructs bowel activity can contribute to your weight. Chances are, at some point you've heard that, at the time of his death, John Wayne had over 40 pounds of impacted waste in his colon. Although this is in fact an urban legend, the average American by the time they're 30 years old is estimated to have *10 to 15 pounds of hard, impacted fecal matter* caked along the sides of their bowels or in distended areas of the intestinal tract.

That's a lifetime worth of toxins festering away inside the body. If healthy, consistent bowel movements and regular colon cleansing had eliminated the bulk of these toxins, this situation could have been prevented. Toxic residue accumulates over time, and can lead to a swelling in the intestinal walls. This is merely one of the more obvious symptoms of bowel toxemia, or, as we've been calling it, a toxic colon.

It's easy to see the difference between a healthy and an unhealthy colon. The colon shown in Figure 1 on page 4 is obviously healthy and full of life. Unfortunately, the average colon looks a lot more like an unhealthy, toxin-ridden colon in Figure 2 on page 8, with a variety of disease conditions shown for purposes of illustration.

It may sound silly, but listening to nature when it calls is one of the most important things you can do to help maintain your health. Many people are so busy that they simply won't take the time to have a bowel movement when the urge strikes them. Some people prefer to have bowel movements only at home, and will go to great lengths to avoid using a public restroom while at work or out running errands. But if the delay is too long, or too frequent, ignoring the urge to go can lead to constipation and fecal compaction, both of which contribute to toxic buildup in the colon.

Constipation and fecal impaction can also cause stool transit time to slow down. *Transit time* is basically a simple way of saying "the time it takes our bodies to process food and pass waste."

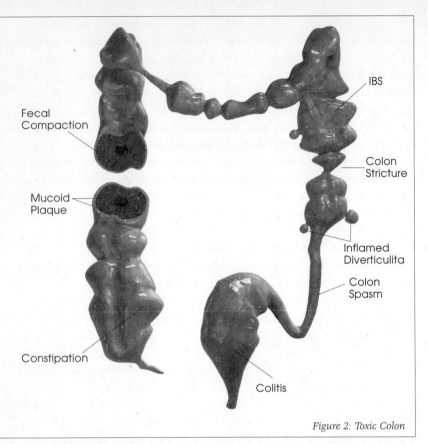

Fecal Compaction

Mucoid Plaque

Constipation

IBS

Colon Stricture

Inflamed Diverticulita

Colon Spasm

Colitis

Figure 2: Toxic Colon

If undigested food hangs out in the body for too long, the proteins putrefy, the carbohydrates ferment, and the fats turn rancid. This changes the compounds in the food from good to bad. This rotten food collects inside the colon, making regular bowel movements increasingly difficult.

How Do All These "Toxins" Cause Disease?

Have you ever noticed that some people who smoke, who drink, and who never exercise sometimes live long, disease-free lives, despite all? And that sometimes people who make healthy choices, and who eat balanced vegetarian diets, develop illnesses? Does this make any sense?

Everybody has their own individual tolerance for the chemicals and other substances entering the body, depending on factors such as lifestyle, environmental exposure, stress levels, and even genetics. This is known as the body's *"toxic threshold,"* or the amount of toxic abuse that the body can handle on a daily basis before it starts to break down.

To give you an example of how everything we discuss in this book contributes to a toxic colon, and to indicate how important regular intestinal cleansing is, I've devised a chart. Now, keep in mind that there's no way of knowing exactly how many toxins from each category you're taking in every day, but I've done my best to calculate the risk factors and to average the toxins in each category.

These calculations are at the lower end of the scale. *Most people consume two to three times the amount I have listed below, every 24 hours.* Depending on your everyday environmental exposure and the personal choices you make regarding your health, these numbers could be greater than the examples below, or (if you're lucky) less than them.

This may seem like a huge, almost unimaginable number of toxins. And it is. *But a single bag of a synthetic sugar substitute can contain over 10,000 toxic molecules.*

Don't worry, I will go over each type of toxin in detail in Chapters 6 and 7 and tell you exactly what you need to do to either eliminate or replace them.

If your body can only handle 1 million toxins daily, but you are exposed to over 1.8 million toxins every day, your body must work extra hard, expending much-needed energy, to process or store these compounds. In essence, your body is overwhelmed every 24 hours, day after day.

Now can you see what's happening in your body 365 days a year?

I like to give the example of "1 million," because it's a nice, round, scary number, but this is actually a really low number. The combination of *all* the toxins listed is directly exposed to your intestinal lining every day and, if they are not eliminated, they leak into the blood, initiating the disease process.

In Part 2 of this book I will explain how disease comes about through a toxic colon. I'll have to cover some pretty shocking things there, but my goal for the book is to teach you how to prevent disease, how to clean your intestines properly, and how to eliminate or help eliminate disease from your body so that you can go on to live a longer, healthier, happier life. I believe you need to know how to address and remove the root cause of health problems, as well as understand any current symptoms you may have.

We do have other options available to us, instead of totally relying on our medical system. We can refuse to take a prescription drug, or decline undergoing surgery, for everything we suffer from. Drugs or

Examples of Potential Daily Toxin Intake

Let's say your body can only handle 1 million toxins every 24 hours before breaking down. Every 24 hours, you will be exposed to approximately the following number of toxins:

TOXINS FROM FOOD: 325,000
Examples: white flour; sugar in desserts; hormones and antibiotics; soy; pesticides; genetically modified foods; cooked, boxed, canned, and processed foods; MSG; hydrogenated oils; fast foods; and more.

TOXINS FROM BEVERAGES: 160,000
Examples: Pasteurized milk; soft drinks, diet drinks, energy drinks, and sports drinks; juice concentrates; coffee; alcohol; refined sugars, artificial sweeteners, artificial colorings; and more.

TOXINS FROM AIR: 200,000
Examples: Fossil fuels, benzene, smoke, chemtrail residue, paint outgassing, carpet outgassing, pet dander, mold and mildew, dust mites, air fresheners, cleaning supplies, and many more.

TOXINS FROM WATER: 150,000
Examples: Arsenic, fluoride, chlorine, prescription drug residue, pesticides, rocket fuel (perchlorate), bisphenol-A (toxin from plastic water bottles), C8 (chemical used to make Teflon), bacteria, parasites, and many others.

TOXINS FROM PRESCRIPTION DRUGS: 180,000
Examples: Aluminum, mercury, chemotherapy, butchered animal parts, synthetic chemicals, liver-toxic glues, fillers, binders, artificial colorings, spermicides, synthetic hormones, vaccines, and more.

TOXINS FROM MICROBES (PARASITES): 525,000
Examples: Bacteria, yeast, fungus, worms, amoebas, and viruses (all of which live off a host organism—*you*, in this case). These organisms consume your vital nutrients and then "go to the bathroom" in your system, secreting massive amounts of harmful acids and toxic waste.

TOXINS FROM PHYSICAL AND EMOTIONAL STRESS: 200,000
Examples: Depression, anxiety, fear, and negative emotions—all cause the body to oversecrete stress hormones and other compounds, in an attempt to balance these conditions. This is dangerous, because the body actually damages itself.

TOXINS FROM HEAVY METALS: 130,000
Examples: Cookware, deodorant, fish, mercury dental fillings, cosmetics, aluminum cans, food, water, light bulbs, many herbal supplements, toothpaste, vaccines, paints, and many more.

TOXINS FROM RADIATION (CAUSES CELL DAMAGE AND DEATH)
Examples: Microwave cooking, x-rays, fault lines (geopathic stress), power lines, cell phones, computers, household appliances, fluorescent lighting, hair dryers, irradiated foods, and more.

THIS IS A TOTAL OF: 1,870,000 TOXINS EVERY 24 HOURS!

surgery never address the root cause of the condition in the first place. And that's why I wrote this book. I want you to understand why we have such a preponderance of degenerative diseases and toxic colons today. The reason is a combination of factors directly related to the environment to which you expose yourself. It's not one particular toxin that causes disease—such as only smoking, or only drinking, or only eating badly. *It's a combination of many different factors caused by too many toxins coming in—and not enough going out.*

I believe the colon is the most neglected organ in the body, perhaps due to embarrassment or lack of knowledge regarding its importance in the hierarchy of our own health concerns. Nevertheless, the colon usually does not receive as much attention as our other organs. This, despite the fact that the colon is every bit as vital to life as our other organs and, in fact, it can be the determining factor between our feeling great or our living a life plagued by illness and fatigue.

Now that you know that your body can handle only about 1 million toxins every day, and that these toxins enter your body through the intestines, let's take a deeper look at some of the more common intestinal conditions.

CHAPTER 2

Conditions of a Toxic Colon

In this chapter I will briefly explain some of the more common conditions caused by the accumulation of colon toxins. In the previous chapter I touched on some of these toxins and told you how the toxins you take in every day cause these disorders. I cover these toxins in great detail in Part 2.

At this point you might be thinking that you do not have anything wrong with your bowel. Most people think that, but please read on—you may be greatly surprised.

Common Bowel Conditions Caused by Everyday Toxin Exposure

What, exactly, can happen when you don't regularly cleanse your intestines and colon? Any number of things. As you read this chapter, some of them will be all too familiar to you—and you'll be glad to find out how to tackle them with consistent, safe, and healthy treatments. Other conditions may surprise you, though they may negatively affect the health of your family members or friends; you should know about them in case they turn up in your own body, as well.

Constipation

The U.S. Department of Health and Human Services has openly admitted that "over 90%" of Americans are walking around with "clogged colons."

Constipation is the most common bowel condition worldwide. It is so prevalent and widespread that it should be listed as an epidemic. Whether you think so or not, you are constipated. The shocking truth is that the medical definition of constipation is dead wrong.

The medical definition of constipation: The passage of small amounts of hard, dry bowel movements, usually fewer than three times per week.

What happened to eliminations numbering "three times per day"? Just look at the animal kingdom—birds, horses, cows, anything that lives on and eats from the earth (apart from humans). These animals have multiple bowel movements every day—sometimes more than 10 per day. But when is the last time you saw a cow constipated and straining in the field, or a horse in a corral, or a bird in the bush? Your own bowel habits should be no different. We should be having multiple bowel movements daily.

*The **real** definition of constipation:* If you are not having a minimum of two, soft, easy-to-pass bowel movements daily, then in my professional opinion you are constipated. If your stools are soft, do not have a foul odor, and pass easily, and if you pass them at least two times per day, then I would say that you are not constipated. But remember, this does not mean that you don't still have pounds of hard, compacted fecal matter throughout your entire intestinal tract.

WHAT ARE THE SYMPTOMS OF CONSTIPATION?

A lot of people who suffer from constipation feel that they have incomplete bowel evacuations. This feeling causes them to strain even more, which can lead to anal tears or hemorrhoids, or both, over time. Other constipation symptoms include increased bowel sounds, fatigue, bad breath, and skin blemishes.

Do people step away from you when you are talking to them close up? You might have bad breath, most of the time. And you might be surprised to learn that *bad breath* is a symptom of constipation, for it is commonly overlooked. Yet it makes perfect sense, when you think about it. After all, the mouth and stomach are connected. A digestive tract that's sluggish due to constipation can cause the mouth to have a putrid odor. This is due to gases rising up from the stomach and lingering in the mouth. Plus, halitosis is a signal that your body is trying to tell you something. Your body hopes you will smell this odor and address the cause by cleansing your system and eliminating the toxins from your environment. Your body will always give you signs and signals when something is wrong. You just need to listen and pay attention.

Skin eruptions or blemishes can also be signs of a toxic colon and constipation. Constipation can cause acne and worsen existing acne conditions. Many people never realize that the skin is a major organ responsible for eliminating waste. If the liver and kidneys become overwhelmed by toxic substances that need to be evacuated from the body, the skin does its best to bail them out by helping in this process.

Individuals who are constipated are backed up with fecal matter, and it is impossible for the skin to remove such matter. However, the epidermis (the outer layer of the skin) can show signs of attempting to rid the body of toxins by becoming inflamed or breaking out.

HOW DOES REGULAR COLON CLEANSING HELP CONSTIPATION?

o Cleans the encrusted buildup from the walls of the intestinal lining, thereby increasing the absorption of vital nutrients that your body needs

o Helps promote stools that are passed more frequently

o Helps promote better consistency and greater volume of stool

o Helps in the formation of stools that are easier to pass without straining

o Greatly reduces the chances of developing constipation-related diseases

o Reduces the number of toxins absorbed into the blood

o Improves bowel transit time

Many people ignore their constipation, or are not so blissfully unaware of it, because they have lived with it for so long. They have forgotten how it feels to be healthy, and to have normal bowel movements. Ignoring constipation is not a good idea. Doing so can put your health in danger. Living with constipation should never be a daily routine for anyone. Constipation is one of many precursors for all bowel disease as well as for many diseases that develop elsewhere in the body.

Untreated constipation can lead to extremely serious problems, such as bowel obstruction, which is characterized by a tender stomach and vomiting. It can also lead to episodes of diarrhea. Many people who experience diarrhea don't understand that it is caused by being constipated. What's called "paradoxical diarrhea" occurs when soft stools pass around the impacted matter lodged in the colon. X-rays are usually performed during these stages of constipation to reveal the location of the impacted fecal matter in the bowel. Surgery is sometimes required in severe cases of constipation.

The good news is that when people keep their intestines and colon cleansed, they do not have to suffer from constipation any longer.

Irritable Bowel Syndrome

Look around you—one in five American adults has symptoms of irritable bowel syndrome. IBS, or irritable bowel syndrome, also called "spastic colon," is characterized by mild but persistent problems of the gut. Its symptoms may even pose long-term danger to the colon. IBS can seriously interfere with the everyday lives of people afflicted by the condition. In most cases, however, the triggers and symptoms of IBS can be managed through a combination of dietary and lifestyle changes, along with consistent colon cleansing.

WHAT ARE THE SYMPTOMS OF IBS?

Abdominal discomfort and bloating are the most commonly reported complaints of people with irritable bowel syndrome. A number of other symptoms are also regularly documented. Some people are constipated and report straining to have a bowel movement, as well as having difficulty passing anything at all. Other people experience diarrhea, which is of course on the opposite end of the spectrum. Still others report alternating bouts of constipation and diarrhea.

In addition to physical symptoms, people with IBS frequently suffer from depression and anxiety, which can worsen symptoms. Similarly, the symptoms associated with IBS can, by themselves, cause a person to feel depressed and anxious. So the cycle repeats itself.

Medical science has not yet identified the specific cause of IBS. Some theories suggest that many people with IBS may be overly sensitive to certain things that would not bother a normal person's digestive system. Stress, large meals, intestinal gas, medicines, certain foods, coffee, milk, and alcohol are some of many stimuli that may affect and irritate the colon.

But I'll let you in on a little secret. Do you really want to know what causes IBS? I'm sure you've already guessed by now. It's the accumulation of toxins, and their constant bombardment, in the colon.

DID YOU KNOW? Over 90 percent of your body's *serotonin* is actually housed in the digestive tract. Current research suggests that some people with IBS may have digestive systems containing abnormal levels of that chemical hormone, a neurotransmitter that helps regulate emotions, body temperature, sexuality, and appetite. This can lead to increased abdominal discomfort and problems with bowel movements.

WHO IS AT RISK FOR IBS?

Irritable bowel syndrome occurs more than twice as often in women than in men, and tends to begin in early adulthood. Genetics may play a role, because many people who suffer from IBS have relatives who also have the condition.

It can be quite difficult to diagnose this condition, because a doctor doing a standard colon examination will find no precise indications of it. Instead, the doctor is forced to rely entirely on the medical history provided by the patient.

HOW DOES REGULAR COLON CLEANSING BOTH HELP AND PREVENT IBS?

o Eliminates built-up toxins and rids the intestinal walls of yeast and bad bacteria. It sets the stage for a fresh, new balance of healthy gut flora. People with IBS lack good bacteria in the bowels.

o Helps relieve stress and anxiety, which contribute to flare-ups of IBS.

o Helps calm the overactive nerves in the intestinal tract, thereby reducing inflammation associated with IBS.

o Lessens transit time, reducing the constant irritation of the bowel lining.

o Helps relieve abdominal cramping, bloating, gas, and pain associated with IBS.

Diverticular Disease

As we grow older, the lining of our intestines becomes thin and loses its elasticity, just as our skin does. Small pouches of tissue known as diverticula bulge through these weak spots. One in 10 middle-aged Americans has at least a few of these pouches in their intestines. Some researchers estimate that as much as 50 percent of the elderly population has them. The condition of having these small pouches is referred to as diverticulosis.

For the most part, the condition goes unnoticed. But in about one-fifth of the cases, the pouches become irritated or infected; this is referred to as diverticulitis. The infected pouches can make passing a bowel movement very painful, which can lead to constipation and other complications.

WHAT ARE THE SYMPTOMS OF DIVERTICULAR DISEASE?

Many people with diverticulosis experience no symptoms whatsoever, though some report mild cramps, constipation, and bloating. Diverticulitis, by contrast, is characterized by abdominal pain (especially along the left side), cramping, constipation, fever, nausea, vomiting, and chills.

Since these symptoms are associated with a number of other digestive disorders, diverticular disease can be difficult to diagnose. To determine whether that's the problem, a doctor will first ask a series of questions about the patient's bowel habits, diet, and other potential risk factors. A digital rectal examination may also be performed. Other methods include x-rays, ultrasound, CT scanning, colonoscopy, and sigmoidoscopy.

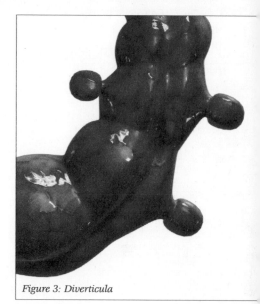

Figure 3: Diverticula

Untreated, the disease can lead to a number of serious complications, most of which arise when a portion of the colon wall becomes torn or perforated. As a result of this tearing, toxic waste matter can leak from the intestine into the abdominal cavity. This can cause serious health problems such as the following:

- Abscesses—Infections in the abdomen that become "walled off"
- Peritonitis—An infection of the abdominal cavity that is very painful and life threatening
- Obstructions—Blockages in the intestine
- Fistulas—A connection between two organs or between an organ and the skin

DOCTOR'S NOTE: Every year, diverticular disease accounts for some 576,000 hospitalizations in the United States.

WHO IS AT RISK FOR DIVERTICULAR DISEASE?

Diverticular disease becomes more common as people age. In fact, almost 70 percent of the population will develop diverticular disease by the age of 85. Again, the constant bombardment of colon toxins, especially from food, contributes to an increased risk for developing this condition.

HOW DOES REGULAR COLON CLEANSING BOTH HELP AND PREVENT DIVERTICULAR DISEASE?

o Eliminates built-up toxins that may be stored in diverticular pouches.

o Rids the intestinal walls of the bad bacteria that cause diverticulitis (producing infection and inflammation).

o Prevents the diverticuli from becoming infected and swollen.

o Helps relieve constipation, which contributes to the development of diverticular disease.

o Strengthens the intestinal walls, preventing thinning, weakening, and bulging.

o Lessens transit time, reducing exposure of the bowel lining to toxic acids.

o Helps restore proper bowel function, which reduces the chances of developing diverticulitis.

Celiac Disease

About 2 million people in America have celiac disease, a number that continues to rise. Celiac disease is caused by a genetic intolerance to *gluten*, a plant protein found mostly in cereal grains. When a person with celiac disease eats foods that contain gluten, their immune system responds by attacking their small intestine. The damage caused by the immune system can disrupt the intestine's ability to absorb nutrients, which causes afflicted individuals to become malnourished regardless of the quantity of the foods they eat.

Although most doctors would never tell you this, if you're suffering from celiac disease, then you almost certainly have some form of stone-related liver/gallbladder malfunction. This is due to the fact that all the nutrients (including glutens) that the small intestine absorbs are eventually deposited in either the liver or the gallbladder. (It is not uncommon to expel 100 to 500 stones after performing a good cleanse of the liver or gallbladder.)

WHAT ARE THE SYMPTOMS OF CELIAC DISEASE?

Many people with celiac disease show no symptoms at all. This is especially dangerous, because they are unaware of the damage going on inside their bodies. If symptoms do surface, they can vary substantially from person to person, but may include abdominal pain, gas, bloating, diarrhea, weight changes, fatigue, joint pain, tingling in the legs, muscle cramps, seizures, menstrual and fertility problems, mouth sores, tooth discoloration, skin irritation, and osteoporosis. The damage caused to the small intestine, combined with poor nutrient absorption, can also put people with celiac disease at an increased risk for developing colon cancer.

WHO IS AT RISK FOR CELIAC DISEASE?

Research on celiac disease is somewhat scarce, compared to other types of bowel disease. It has been observed, however, that Caucasian people, particularly those of European descent, are more likely to develop the illness. Celiac disease is one of the most common genetic diseases in the Western world. In many regions of Europe, it affects 1 in some 250 to 300 people. Celiac disease is almost never diagnosed among African or Asian peoples.

Until recently the incidence of celiac disease appeared to be much lower in the United States, though recent studies suggest that the disease is equally common among Americans of European decent—it's just astonishingly underdiagnosed.

HOW DOES REGULAR COLON CLEANSING HELP CELIAC DISEASE?

o Eliminates built-up toxins in the bowel and keeps the intestinal walls clean.

o Helps relieve the pressure on the liver and gallbladder, reducing the number of stones formed.

o Strengthens the intestinal walls, preventing leakage of toxins back into the liver.

o Lessens transit time, reducing exposure of the bowel lining to gluten.

DOCTOR'S NOTE: The most straightforward method of dealing with celiac disease is to completely remove gluten from your diet. Celiac disease is a lifelong autoimmune intestinal disorder, found in individuals who are genetically susceptible. Damage to the mucosal surface of the small intestine is caused by an immunologically toxic reaction to the ingestion of gluten and interferes with the absorption of nutrients. A large percentage of people with the disease are often relieved of it by regularly cleansing their colon, liver, and gallbladder.

Inflammatory Bowel Disease

IBD, or inflammatory bowel disease, is one name for two quite similar diseases, both of which cause destructive swelling and inflammation in the intestinal tract. The two conditions, *Crohn's disease* and *ulcerative colitis*, are characterized by nearly identical symptoms, which makes it difficult for even trained professionals to distinguish between them. Up to 20 percent of people with ulcerative colitis have a family member or relative with ulcerative colitis or Crohn's disease.

These diseases can have especially gruesome effects in young children, because one of the hallmark symptoms of both of them is persistently bloody diarrhea. This can quickly lead to anemia, malnourishment, and ultimately even stunted development of what should be a growing mind and body.

CROHN'S DISEASE

Severe inflammation and swelling deep within the lining of the digestive tract characterize Crohn's disease. This swelling can be so painful that it forces the intestines to expel waste prematurely as diarrhea. While the condition most commonly affects the intestines, it can also affect other portions of the digestive tract, such as the mouth and stomach (and yes, the mouth is at one end of the digestive tract). In some cases, multiple sections of the digestive tract can be inflamed even while the areas between them remain perfectly healthy.

HOW DOES REGULAR COLON CLEANSING BOTH HELP AND PREVENT CROHN'S DISEASE?

o Eliminates built-up toxins and cleanses the intestinal walls.

o May prevent and reduce the inflammation of intestinal tissue.

o Strengthens the intestinal walls, reinforcing weak spots that could be susceptible to Crohn's.

o Sets up a hospitable environment for the natural balance of probiotic strains needed to help repair the intestinal lining.

o Lessens transit time, which reduces exposure of the bowel lining to toxins.

o Helps restore proper bowel function, lessening the possibility of multiple surgeries.

What Are the Symptoms of Crohn's Disease?

The two most widely reported symptoms of Crohn's disease are diarrhea and abdominal pain on the right side. Other symptoms may include weight loss, arthritis, skin problems, fever, and rectal bleeding (chronic bleeding can lead to anemia).

Crohn's disease is arguably the more severe of the two forms of IBD. Up to 75 percent of those who suffer from it are recommended for surgery at least once. In fact, it's not uncommon for patients to undergo multiple rounds of surgery to remove damaged sections of their intestines in an effort to alleviate the symptoms of the disease. With regular cleansing, though, plus the addition of soil-based probiotics, surgery can be prevented and the intestinal lining can be repaired.

Who Is at Risk for Crohn's Disease?

Crohn's disease is most often diagnosed in people between the ages of 20 and 30. Individuals with relatives who suffer from some form of IBD also run a much greater risk of developing Crohn's. Approximately 20 percent of people coping with Crohn's disease have a close blood relative (most often a brother or sister) with inflammatory bowel disease. Having Jewish ancestry appears to also significantly increase risk, though being African American decreases the risk for this condition.

ULCERATIVE COLITIS

The condition known as ulcerative colitis causes inflammation in the lining of the colon and rectum. The symptoms are similar to those seen in patients suffering from Crohn's disease, though ulcerative colitis does not affect the small intestine, mouth, esophagus, and stomach. A main difference between the two conditions is the depth of inflammation in the intestinal wall.

In Crohn's, all layers of the digestive tissue are susceptible. With colitis, by contrast, only the surface of the intestinal lining is affected. Colitis completely destroys portions of the lining and leaves behind open sores, or ulcers. These ulcers continuously leak blood and toxic pus back into the digestive system, which can further inflame the bowel and lead to more ulcers. Another vicious cycle. In a lot of ways, the two conditions are like a fire that constantly pours gasoline on itself.

HOW DOES REGULAR COLON CLEANSING BOTH HELP AND PREVENT ULCERATIVE COLITIS?

o Eliminates built-up toxins and keeps the intestinal walls clean of toxic material.

o Reduces the acid concentrations in the intestinal lining, preventing the development of ulcerated tissue.

o Helps clean existing ulcerations, and shortens healing time of ulcerated tissue.

o Lessens transit time, which reduces the constant irritation of the ulcers by hard, compacted fecal matter.

o Helps restore proper mucus secretion, hereby lubricating the walls and creating less irritation and friction around ulcerated sites.

Abdominal pain and bloody diarrhea are most commonly experienced conditions of ulcerative colitis. Sufferers also sometimes report fatigue, weight loss, change in appetite, skin lesions, and fever. Seemingly unrelated afflictions such as osteoporosis, arthritis, liver disease, and eye inflammation have been reported, yet medical doctors still aren't exactly sure why. Drugs are usually prescribed to help control the symptoms of colitis for as long as possible. Unfortunately, the available drugs aren't especially effective, and, sad to say, about one-third of all patients diagnosed with the disease eventually have their colons removed, with the changes in lifestyle that entails. Most of these surgeries are unnecessary, and in my view the majority could be avoided with regular cleansing.

Who Is at Risk for Ulcerative Colitis?

People of Caucasian or Jewish ancestry between the ages of 15 and 30 have a higher risk of developing colitis. As with Crohn's disease, approximately 20 percent of individuals with ulcerative colitis have relatives diagnosed with IBD.

Colon Polyps

Sometimes featured (or, alarmingly, even graphically shown) in the news when celebrities or political figures have them removed, colon polyps are small growths of tissue. They're something like a large mole or wart that develops along the internal lining of the colon. Like real skin moles, small polyps aren't usually dangerous. But since some larger polyps can eventually develop into cancer, most doctors will remove polyps of any size that they encounter when doing a colonoscopy of a patient. Unlike most diverticula polyps, which don't develop into colon cancer, most internal colon polyps will.

WHAT ARE THE SYMPTOMS OF COLON POLYPS?

Typically, people with colon polyps don't notice any symptoms. The polyps, therefore, can be sneaky. Many people first find out that they have them during a colonoscopy or sigmoidoscopy checkup. But it's not uncommon for people to experience symptoms such as constipation, diarrhea, and blood in the stool.

WHO IS AT RISK FOR GETTING COLON POLYPS?

Your chances of developing polyps increase if:

- You're over 40 years old

- You have previously had polyps

- A relative or family member has had polyps

- A family member or relative has had colorectal cancer

- You eat a high-fat diet

- You smoke, or you drink alcohol

- You don't regularly exercise

- You are 15 or more pounds overweight

- You do not regularly cleanse your liver, gallbladder, and intestinal tract

WHAT TREATMENT OPTIONS ARE AVAILABLE?

The most common method of treating colon polyps is for a doctor to remove them during your colonoscopy (since they can be seen by a tiny camera during that procedure, which is attached to an instrument that can snip off the polyps). The polyps are then tested for malignancy. But once again this addresses only the symptom, not the cause. If a polyp was there before, what is to prevent it from growing back, just like a fingernail or your hair? In fact, in the majority of cases polyps *do* grow back.

Keeping up with a healthy diet and maintaining a sufficient exercise routine, plus avoiding as many colon toxins as possible, are good ways to reduce the chances of developing polyps. I also recommend regularly cleansing of the colon, which will help keep the intestinal lining free of toxic compaction that could give rise to polyps that could turn cancerous.

HOW DOES REGULAR COLON CLEANSING BOTH HELP AND PREVENT COLON POLYPS?

- Eliminates built-up toxins and cleanses the intestinal walls of toxic material, reducing the chances of polyp development.

- Lessens transit time, which minimizes the constant irritation to the intestinal lining.

- Reduces the size of polyps, which reduces the risk of developing colon cancer.

- Helps eliminate *Candida* and fungus suspected of initiating polyp growth.

Colon Cancer

Also known as colorectal cancer (because it involves both colon and rectum), colon cancer is one of the most common cancers in the United States, and is spreading around the globe at alarming rates. *Approximately half the cases of colorectal cancer result in death.* That's a pretty scary statistic, when you know that practically all these cases could have been prevented.

Normally, colon cancer develops when benign colon polyps become cancerous and go on to damage the delicate intestinal tissue.

WHAT ARE THE SYMPTOMS OF COLON CANCER?

Polyps often go undetected, since most people suffer from few symptoms, or none. It's frightening but true that the same is the case with colon cancer caused by cancerous polyps. As the polyps slowly develop into cancer, many individuals have no discomfort or other symptoms. However, many people do experience one or more of the

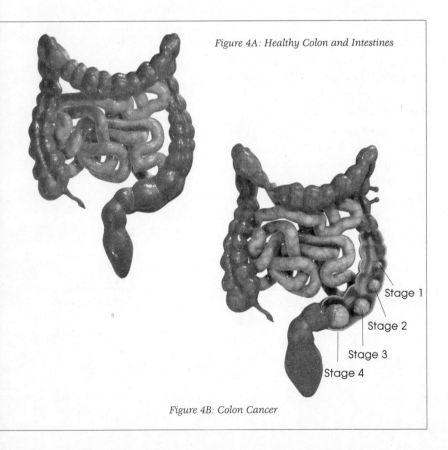

Figure 4A: Healthy Colon and Intestines

Stage 1
Stage 2
Stage 3
Stage 4

Figure 4B: Colon Cancer

following symptoms: bloody stools, abdominal pain, alternating bouts of diarrhea and constipation, weight loss, changes in appetite, anemia, fatigue, or pale complexion.

WHO IS AT RISK FOR COLON CANCER?

Everyone is at risk for developing colon cancer. Factors that may elevate your risk for developing colon cancer include having polyps or inflammatory bowel disease, having preexisting cancer in another part of the body (particularly the breast), and having relatives who developed colorectal cancer. Females over the age of 40 are also slightly more likely to develop colorectal cancer—it's estimated that 1 in 26 women, as opposed to 1 in 27 men, will suffer from the disease at some point in their life. The biggest risk factor for you, however, is the amount of daily toxins you expose yourself to.

Remember the toxic threshold we talked about in Chapter 1? Reducing these daily toxins from your environment is the easiest way to prevent the development of colon cancer.

People who are diagnosed in the early stages of the disease are much more likely to recover. Late detection of malignant polyps is one of the main reasons that colorectal cancer accounts for an estimated one in five cancer deaths in the United States.

My personal and professional belief is that all cancers of the body start from toxic overload in the liver or in the intestines, coupled with negative emotional stressors.

HOW DOES COLON CLEANSING BOTH HELP AND PREVENT COLON CANCER?

o Eliminates built-up toxins and rids the intestinal walls of toxic material, reducing the chances that polyps will become malignant.

o Lessens transit time, which minimizes irritation to the intestinal lining. This helps prevent the formation of cancer-causing polyps.

o Decreases the size of polyps, which reduces the risk of developing colon cancer.

o Helps balance intestinal pH levels, thereby reducing the acidic environment needed for cancerous tissue to develop.

o Prevents chronic fermentation in the bowels, reducing the levels of glucose. Glucose is the main source of food for cancerous tissue.

CHAPTER 3

How Healthy Is Your Colon?

The condition of your internal plumbing is not a particularly pleasant topic, so most of us don't give much thought to how healthy our colon is, or pay close attention to our bowel movements. And the subject doesn't exactly come up much in conversation, either. This is totally understandable, but if you're truly serious about restoring and maintaining your health, you have to start paying attention to your colon by monitoring your bowel movements. You have to *investigate what you eliminate*.

In most health matters, it's hard to know exactly what's "normal." After all, everyone's body operates a little differently, and we're all exposed to different environments and enjoy different diets and lifestyles. Nevertheless, there *are* some general indicators that you can use to check for what I'll call normal, healthy bowel movements.

Stools should typically be soft and easy to pass. If you experience bloating, gas, bad breath, skin blemishes, hard or pellet-like stools, or fewer than three bowel movements daily—or if you have to strain with bowel movements even once or twice a week—then there's a good chance that your colon is not healthy. Ideally, stools should be brown or golden brown, be shaped like link-sausage, and have a texture similar to peanut butter.

Unfortunately, many of us consistently experience abnormal bowel movements without even realizing it. Constipation and diarrhea have become two of the most common conditions afflicting practically everyone in the world. They have become so normal, in fact, that we don't see them for what they really are—a cry for help from our colons.

Analyze Your Stool

To enable health care professionals to better diagnose these conditions, as well as others that affect the bowels, a standardized system of measurement was created to assess the size, shape, and consistency of *stool* (a word meaning a discharge of fecal matter, derived from an Old English word for *chair, seat,* and *throne,* where most people sit when having a bowel movement).

The Bristol Stool Scale, shown on page 30, was developed in 1997 by a small team of gastroenterologists at the University of Bristol, in the U.K. It was designed to be a general measurement system used by health care professionals to evaluate the consistency or form of stools. This scale is a medical tool designed to classify bowel movements (as they appear in toilet water) into seven distinct categories. A direct correlation exists between the form the stool takes and the amount of time it has spent in the colon before being eliminated.

You don't have to be a digestive health expert to benefit from the Bristol Stool Scale. You can easily use it at home to analyze everyday bowel movements. The scale can also be a useful tool for tracking changes inside your digestive system that can alert you that your colon isn't functioning the way it's supposed to.

According to current medical science, types 3 and 4 stools, if passed at least once every three days, qualify as "normal." I strongly disagree with this. I firmly believe that you should have *at least two type 3 or type 4 bowel movements every single day of your life.*

In general, if you're constipated, your stools are categorized as either type 1 or type 2. Some estimate that over 90 percent of Americans live with the daily discomfort of passing types 1 and 2 stools. This trend is sure to continue if lifestyle changes aren't made soon across a wide spectrum of people.

Those who are suffering from diarrhea pass types 5, 6, or 7 stools on an uncomfortably frequent basis. Every year, *272 million*

Americans (that's almost every one of us) get diarrhea one or more times per year.

BE AWARE OF THE CONDITION OF YOUR STOOL

You should keep an eye on your stool every day or so. Mucus in the stool can be either a symptom of digestive problems or a result of a successful colon cleansing. Knowing the difference between the two depends largely on the circumstances. Either way, it's important to be able to recognize mucus in your stool.

Mucus can also be caused by eating unhealthy foods, dairy products, or foods to which you may be allergic. With food allergens, the intestinal wall produces extra mucus to protect itself. Since most people follow unhealthy diets, it's not unusual for the digestive system to produce excess mucus.

How Do I Identify Mucus in My Stool?

Mucus is fairly easy to identify. It can be white, yellow, or clear in color. In all cases, however, it has a light jelly-like consistency. Mucus may cover the entire surface of the bowel movement or may appear as small particles that are sometimes mistaken for worms.

Seeing mucus in your stool isn't necessarily a sign of a problem. In fact, the large intestine naturally produces protective mucus to trap foreign particles and move waste through the colon. Since the mucus serves to protect your digestive system, it's not unusual to find increased amounts of it when you are suffering from constipation or diarrhea.

When Is Mucus a Bad Sign?

If you experience mucus only occasionally, you shouldn't be too concerned about it. But if you produce mucus for more than a few weeks, or if it's accompanied by an unusually foul smell or bleeding, you should consult with a health care professional as soon as possible, because it could be a symptom of serious health problems.

DOCTOR'S NOTE: Some foods produce more mucus than others. Ayurvedic medicine calls such foods *kapha* foods. (*Kapha* comes from a Sanskrit word meaning "phlegm.") Examples are dairy, wheat, sugar, foods in the night shade family (such as potatoes, tomatoes, bell peppers, and peppers), bananas, oranges, tangerines, and grapefruits. They are said to aggravate allergies. Even if you have no apparent food allergies you can have extra mucus drainage from eating such foods.

TAKE NOTE IF YOU HAVE STOOL OF A DIFFERENT COLOR

Green Stools: Bowel movements that are green can be caused by several factors, primarily related to dietary issues. In most cases, green stools are harmless, though they could indicate a symptom of a digestive disorder. If you can attribute a green bowel movement to something you ate, then it's not a cause for concern. But if it occurs repeatedly, you may want to check it out with your health care professional. Bile is green in color and is secreted by the liver directly into the small intestine or stored in the gallbladder. It is released to break down fats. As normal stool forms from the small intestine to the colon, it changes from green to yellow to brown. When transit time is lessened because of an underlying condition, your bowel movements can take on a green color. It is also normal for breastfed infants to have green-looking stools.

> **MUCUS-COVERED STOOLS COULD BE A WARNING SIGN FOR:**
>
> o Ulcerative colitis
>
> o Irritable bowel syndrome
>
> o Infection
>
> o Bowel obstruction

White Stools: Stools that are white can indicate trouble with the kidneys or biliary system (consisting of the gallbladder and the ducts that carry bile and other digestive enzymes to the small intestine). Bile is responsible for creating the colors commonly seen in waste matter. If there's a problem with these systems, the bile may not be formulated correctly and a white bowel movement can result. If you produce a bowel movement that is solid white all the way through, it's important to immediately consult with a physician specializing in digestive disorders.

If your body digests food too quickly, you might experience a white bowel movement. In this case, the white color is due to mucus, not bile. If waste passes through your body too fast, the mucus produced by your colon may not be digested before the feces is eliminated.

Although this may not be especially pleasant to do, you can determine the cause of your white bowel movement by soaking the stool in water (say, in a bucket or basin placed in the bathtub, not the toilet; use a slotted spoon to remove it from the toilet). If it is a mucus-covered stool, the white mucus should disintegrate, leaving behind "normal"-looking waste matter. White stools caused by problems with bile production will remain white.

Having a small amount of mucus in your stool is considered normal, since your digestive system naturally produces it to aid in

continued on page 32

BRISTOL STOOL SCALE

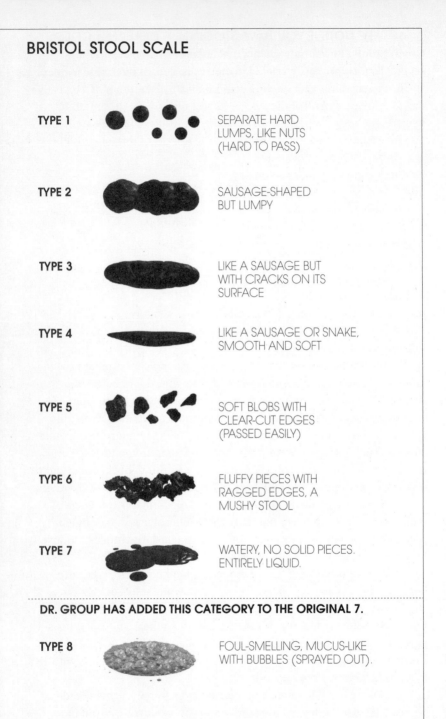

TYPE 1 — SEPARATE HARD LUMPS, LIKE NUTS (HARD TO PASS)

TYPE 2 — SAUSAGE-SHAPED BUT LUMPY

TYPE 3 — LIKE A SAUSAGE BUT WITH CRACKS ON ITS SURFACE

TYPE 4 — LIKE A SAUSAGE OR SNAKE, SMOOTH AND SOFT

TYPE 5 — SOFT BLOBS WITH CLEAR-CUT EDGES (PASSED EASILY)

TYPE 6 — FLUFFY PIECES WITH RAGGED EDGES, A MUSHY STOOL

TYPE 7 — WATERY, NO SOLID PIECES. ENTIRELY LIQUID.

DR. GROUP HAS ADDED THIS CATEGORY TO THE ORIGINAL 7.

TYPE 8 — FOUL-SMELLING, MUCUS-LIKE WITH BUBBLES (SPRAYED OUT).

ANALYZING YOUR STOOL

TYPE 1: *Feces are eliminated as separate, hard lumps, somewhat like nuts.* Type 1 stools spend more time in the colon than any other type, and are generally difficult to pass. Such stools are a sure sign that you're constipated, have toxic conditions in your colon, and need regular intestinal cleansing. Type 1 stools are the most common type among Americans.

TYPE 2: *Stool is shaped like link-sausage, and is bumpy.* These stools indicate that you are constipated, have toxic conditions, and need regular intestinal cleansing.

TYPE 3: *Stool is shaped like sausage, and has cracks in the surface.* Type 3 stools are considered normal.

TYPE 4: Stool is shaped like sausage, and is smooth and soft. Type 4 stools are considered normal.

TYPE 5: *Feces form soft blobs with clear-cut edges* that are easily passed through the system. These stools are classified as soft diarrhea and indicate a possible risk for bowel disease. Type 5 stools also indicate that your colon is toxic and needs regular intestinal cleansing.

TYPE 6: *Stools have fluffy pieces with ragged edges.* These are considered mushy stools, and indicate diarrhea. These stools indicate that your colon is toxic and needs regular intestinal cleansing.

TYPE 7: *Stool is very watery with no solid pieces.* This type of stool has spent the least amount of time in the colon. Type 7 stools indicate severe diarrhea due to cholera or a bacterial or viral infection. See a doctor as soon as possible.

TYPE 8: *Stool is fetid and mucus-like with bubbles (sprayed out).* This indicates excessive intake of alcohol or recreational drugs, or both. Please seek help for your addiction.

(**NOTE:** I've added type 8 stool as an additional category; it is not in the Bristol Stool Scale.)

RECOMMENDATION: If you are experiencing type 1, 2, 5, 6, 7, or 8 stools for longer than three months, I recommend that you perform the "Oxygen Colon Cleanse" as detailed in Chapter 4, followed by three back-to-back liver/gallbladder cleanses (see Resources), and then start slowly eliminating toxins from your daily routine. You may want to see your health care practitioner as well, to determine the root cause of your problem.

TIP: If stools have an extremely foul odor, the cause may be an imbalance of gut bacteria or consumption of too much animal protein. A rancid, foul-smelling odor that lingers for more than five minutes in the bathroom after evacuation is a definite sign that you need to cleanse your colon. Your body is trying to get your attention with that odor— something is wrong inside you. The longer you ignore this, the more damage could occur. Your colon is practically screaming at you. Most people are not taught these critical signs and therefore do not listen to their bodies. Please pay attention to the signs your body gives you.

SOME COMMON CAUSES OF GREEN STOOL

o Food passing through the digestive system too quickly (due to food poisoning, food allergy, or stomach virus)

o Vitamins or supplement containing large amounts of iron

o Eating an excessive amount of sugar

o Consuming too many green, leafy vegetables, and not enough grains

o Using algae or chlorophyll supplements

o During or after a liver/gallbladder cleanse

efficient waste removal. Large amounts of mucus, on the other hand, are not normal and may require action.

Yellow Stools: Stools that are yellow or pale often indicate a condition known as "pale stool." Unless for some reason you ingested massive amounts of food coloring, yellow stool is not normal. If your stool is pale or yellow, then your large intestine, liver, small intestine, or stomach may be affected by a serious condition or disease. Please see a doctor.

Take the Colon Health Self-Test

As with anything related to your health, it's important that you fully know your body before a treatment plan can be put into place, either by yourself alone or in consultation with a health care professional. The following test that you can give yourself will provide you with valuable information about the health of your colon, as well as your personal risk of developing serious intestinal problems.

Simply answer Yes or No to the following questions. Before you know it, you'll have a good idea of the overall condition of your colon. Be honest with yourself. If you find some of the questions difficult to answer, you may first want to keep a journal of your bowel habits and general health for a week or so.

Base your answers over the last 30 days.

1. Do you run out of energy in the afternoon?

2. Do you suffer from occasional headaches?

3. Are you having fewer than 2 or 3 bowel movements daily?

4. Do you have problems concentrating from time to time?

5. Do you experience gas or bloating 1 or more times weekly?

6. Do you get irritable now and then?

7. Do you have difficulty getting a good night's rest?

8. Do you have muscle aches and stiffness?

MORE IRREGULAR COLORS AND FORMS OF STOOL

IF YOUR BOWEL MOVEMENTS ARE...	IT MAY BE DUE TO...
Dark-black and sticky	• Blood in the upper portion of the digestive tract
Very dark-brown	• Recent red wine consumption, an excess of salt, or lack of vegetable intake
Beet-red	• Eating red foods
Superthin, resembling a ribbon	• Polyp development in the colon
Greasy looking	• Insufficient intake of nutrients

9. Do you eat red meat more than 2 times per week?

10. Do you eat fried foods in more than 2 meals per week?

11. Do you drink less than ½ gallon of purified water daily?

12. Do you have problems controlling your weight?

13. Do you exercise less than 3 times weekly?

14. Do you suffer from allergies or sinus problems?

15. Do you have bad breath or body odor?

16. Are you unhappy with your current health?

17. Are you currently suffering from any health problems?

18. Do you have hemorrhoids?

19. Is your skin broken, spotted, or blemished in any way?

20. Do you have occasional abdominal pain?

21. Do you have to strain to have a bowel movement?

22. Do your bowel movements have a foul odor?

23. Do you have hard, small, or dry feces 1 or 2 times weekly?

24. Do you notice bright red blood on the toilet paper 1 or more times per month?

25. Do you have painful bowel movements?

26. Do you use a microwave to cook more than 2 meals per week?

27. Do you drink coffee, soft drinks, alcohol, or milk more than 2 times per week?

28. Are you currently taking any prescription medications?

Now count your "Yes" answers. If you answered "Yes" to more than 7 questions, your bowel is not functioning properly. You are most likely over your daily "toxic threshold" of 1 million toxins.

You've now determined the current health of your colon, so you're ready to learn more about the benefits of cleansing. In the next chapter you will find out how my "Oxygen Colon Cleanse" can jump-start your health, get it headed down the right road, and help you maintain a healthy colon for the rest of your life's journey.

CHAPTER 4

The Oxygen Colon Cleanse

By now you've learned about the different types of colon disease, and you know that all acquired disease starts in the intestinal tract and colon. By this point, you also know how healthy or unhealthy your colon actually is. This chapter will present the most effective ways to cleanse your whole intestinal tract, from top to bottom (so to speak!). At the end of the chapter I will provide some other highly beneficial methods both for cleansing and for general intestinal health.

Because prevention is the best way to maintain maximum health, the chapters in Part 2 explain in detail how common toxins in your environment affect you each and every day. They also provide ample ways for you to reduce your "toxic threshold" by eliminating these toxins for *good*—and I do mean "good"!—once and for all.

If you're anything like most of the people I help with their colon cleansing, or speak to when I'm speaking at a workshop or a conference, then you're probably overwhelmed by the sheer variety of cleansing options out there. The good news is that more and more people are catching on to the importance of regular intestinal cleansing.

Unfortunately, it also seems that a lot of supplement companies are just out to make a buck off this latest craze.

> **CAUTION:** The majority of the products you find in drugstores, supermarkets, and wholesale clubs, as well as many offered on TV and sold over the Internet, are nothing more than cheaply made concoctions that can lead to even *more* colon toxins. If they're good for anything at all, it's cleaning out your wallet. So be aware and check them out thoroughly before buying.

Before continuing, I want to congratulate you on reading this book. By doing so, you are making a commitment to transform your health. You are also investing in your future, with little financial outlay. In this chapter I'll tell you how to avoid years of misery and frustration—the same misery and frustration that millions of Americans suffer every day because they don't have this seldom-discussed information right in front of them, the way you do right now.

Now, I invite you to relax and picture yourself on a day when you're not having those bothersome symptoms of bloating, gas, fatigue, headaches, and any others that you may experience more often than you'd care to (which is "never"). Imagine a day when you feel self-confident, happy, and full of life, not worrying about a single thing.

Can you see yourself on such a day? (Closing your eyes for a few minutes may help.) What favorite activity are you doing? How healthy and happy do you look? Whom are you spending this time with? Really, isn't a moment like this what life is all about?

You can turn that fantasy into a reality. How would you like to, once and for all, get rid of your health concerns and have a normal, healthy body? Wouldn't you truly feel wonderful if you experienced less stress, less irritation, few sluggish feelings or none—just a content, enjoyable, pain-free, worry-free life?

In my professional career, I've spent years not only helping people like you discover the truth about their health problems, but also teaching them how to feel healthy again—quickly, easily, and naturally without any drugs, surgery, or toxic side effects.

That's why I wrote this book. Frankly, I got sick and tired of seeing people walking around being sick and tired, feeling lousy and insecure about themselves, going through a lifetime of misery—all because no one ever bothered to reveal to them "The Secret to Health," discussed in the Introduction of this book: keeping the colon and body clean.

In fact, since I've been helping people just like you, I've focused a majority of my practice and skills on cleansing the body. To me, there is truly nothing more gratifying than helping people just like you to learn how to live life on their own terms, in a healthier fashion.

But I must warn you that it's in your best interest to act right *now*, because later on, if you put this matter off till a "better day," your condition might deteriorate to the point where I can't help you. Either way, though, I wish you good luck and a bright future, shining in the light of excellent health.

I developed the following cleanse for people who want a deep cleansing of the full intestinal tract and colon. I recommend performing this 6-day cleanse at least three to four times per year, plus following up with regular maintenance cleansing one to two times weekly.

The Oxygen Colon Cleanse

6 Days

This cleanse requires the use of an oxygen-based cleanser. In my professional judgment, such colon cleansers are the safest and most effective. If you would like to jump-start the cleansing process, you may also want to do a colon hydrotherapy session before starting this cleanse.

But before you start the daily cleanse program itself (which begins on page 47), please read the following background section. It explains the supplies needed, the drink recipe proportions, and rationales for the various ingredients. Then you will be ready to start a colon cleanse.

SUPPLIES NEEDED FOR THE OXYGEN COLON CLEANSE

- 6 gallons of distilled water
- 8 ounces of organic, raw, unpasteurized apple cider vinegar (available at most grocery stores or health food stores)
- 3 organic lemons (if you can't find organic or locally grown, then use the best lemons in your supermarket)
- 1 bottle Oxy-Powder®, Homozon, or other high-quality oxygen-based intestinal cleanser
- 1 bottle Latero Flora (Bacillus Laterosporus-BOD strain) or good probiotic formula
- Fresh fruit (preferably organic or locally grown)

- 16 ounces of organic, whole-leaf, cold-pressed aloe vera juice (available at your health food store; I use and recommend R PUR Aloe 18X Concentrate—see the Resources section).

Note: If you purchase an aloe vera juice from your local health food store, make sure it is the highest quality available and has no added sugars; organic is always best.

MAKING THE INTESTINAL CLEANSER DRINK

Try your best to drink 1 gallon of the Intestinal Cleanser every day during the 6-day cleanse. It is best to keep your drink refrigerated throughout the day. If you are not able to finish the gallon by the end of the day, discard what remains and start fresh the following day. Do your best to finish the gallon each day.

RECIPE FOR THE CLEANSER DRINK

- Start with 1 gallon of distilled water.
- Pour out 4 ounces of the distilled water.
- Add 2 tablespoons of organic apple cider vinegar. Shake the ACV well before adding to water.
- Add 2 ounces of *organic* aloe vera juice.
- Add the juice of 1/2 organic lemon.
- Mix well and keep refrigerated.

Why Is Organic Apple Cider Vinegar in the Intestinal Cleanser Drink?

Apple cider vinegar may be one of nature's most potent detoxifiers against a variety of negative health conditions. Created through the fermentation of raw apples within wooden barrels, vinegar from apple cider is extremely acidic (with a pH value of around 2.8; pH is a measure of acidity and alkalinity). Its high acidity may be the key factor in its amazing curative powers.

The greater the purity of the apples used in the fermentation process, the greater the health benefits you will have and the better the detoxifying power of the drink. Only fresh, organically grown apples are used, meaning that they have not been treated with pesticides, fertilized with chemicals, or modified genetically.

Organic apple cider vinegar (or ACV, for short) contains fibrous pectin and the "mother." The latter term refers to a structure of protein filaments clinging together in what looks like a spider's web. It's usually visible floating in the vinegar when held up to the light. You'll see cloudiness within the vinegar that appears like tiny grains or strands. These particles add fiber to the ACV and ensure that you receive the most beneficial components of the original apples—their essential vitamins, minerals, enzymes, and amino acids. Nearly 100 health-promoting substances have been identified in organic apple cider vinegar.

One caution: Most nonorganic brands of ACV undergo pasteurization (that is, are boiled to remove bacteria), as well as filtration and distillation. The result is a product so "refined" that it is nutritionally worthless.

ACV is arguably one of the best all-around detoxifiers for your body's intestinal tract and organs. Once you have detoxified your body, it can begin the process of self-healing from an array of diseases and ailments. This is why it's so important to use only organic ACV—it's the sole way to obtain all the life-promoting enzymes and vitamins needed for proper intestinal detoxification.

ACV also inhibits the growth of harmful yeast, germs, fungi, and bacteria in the intestinal tract, thereby increasing the absorption and utilization of vital nutrients.

Common brands of ACV readily available include Braggs, Solana Gold, and Spectrum. (See the Resources section.)

Why Is Aloe Vera Juice in the Intestinal Cleanser Drink?

Aloe vera juice provides a great many positive health benefits. The structural composition of an aloe vera plant includes the very building blocks of life: essential vitamins and minerals, proteins, polysaccharides, enzymes, and amino acids. Of all the plant species catalogued to date, the aloe vera plant's internal makeup is the most closely related to our own biochemistry.

Aloe vera possesses multiple natural qualities for healing and detoxifying the body. When taken internally, it assists the bowels in flushing out accumulated waste and toxic debris. It can help ease a variety

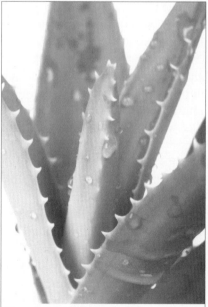

Figure 5: Aloe Vera Plant

of constipation symptoms, improve regularity in bowel movements, and keep the colon clean.

Aloe vera juice (from the whole leaf of the plant) is helpful in alleviating a number of digestive disorders, such as:

- Acid indigestion
- Bloating and gas
- *Candida*
- Colitis
- Constipation
- Diarrhea
- Hemorrhoids
- Irritable bowel syndrome
- Poor appetite
- Sluggish bile production
- Ulcers

Aloe vera contains a large number of mucopolysaccharides (a mouthful, meaning "basic sugars"), which are found in every cell in the body. As mentioned, aloe vera contains essential compounds that enhance nutrient absorption and improve overall digestive function. It also provides many other health benefits, containing more than 200 valuable nutrients.

Aloe vera's tissue regeneration properties work toward rebuilding the tissues of the small and large intestines, the colon, and the stomach. These tissues can become damaged through disease or even extended bouts of constipation. Researchers have found that aloe vera stimulates fibroblasts into constructing new tissue. Aloe polysaccharides improve immune system strength and are highly effective in eliminating toxin-filled waste by boosting internal, natural processes.

One more piece of good news: Aloe vera presents no known side effects and is quite safe. Throughout history, the plant has been universally regarded as nature's gift for treating burns, skin conditions, and digestive difficulties.

The company that makes the aloe I use has mastered the whole-leaf process and created a product it calls Aloe Vera 18X Concentrate. The manufacturer (R PUR Aloe) uses a new, revolutionary whole-leaf, cold process to ensure the product's maximum efficacy and to make sure that it exceeds all International Standards for Aloe Processing (ISAP). And just to let you know, I have no financial interests in the company; I simply think their product is the best.

Traditional methods of refining the aloe vera plant involve a hand-filleting process to remove the gel from the leaf; the leaf is then discarded. Ironically, the largest concentration of the active ingredients, polysaccharides and mucopolysaccharide (Acemannan), are found just beneath the outer surface of the leaf (called the rind). The leaf can be bitter, indigestible, possibly abrasive to your system, and difficult to refine.

The new whole-leaf process employed in the making of R PUR Aloe enables the cellulose to be dissolved and the aloin and aloe emodin to be removed. The entire procedure is done by a cold process, which ensures maximum efficiency and results in a product that is rich in polysaccharides, including mucopolysaccharides (MPS). This is the reason I recommend and use this product in my practice and for myself, as well.

Why Is Lemon Juice in the Intestinal Cleanser Drink?

Drinking fresh-squeezed lemon juice while cleansing provides a superb boost for your colon. Owing to its amazing digestive properties, lemon juice maximizes the Oxygen Colon Cleanse by providing the following benefits:

- Removes impurities from the intestinal tract and body
- Is antiseptic, eliminating the presence of harmful bacteria in the bowel
- Helps alleviate symptoms of heartburn, excess gas, and bloating
- Helps the bowels eliminate waste more efficiently, reducing possible diarrhea or constipation
- Stimulates the liver, for enhanced enzyme production
- Helps create an alkaline condition within the body

The lemon is one of the only "anionic" foods, meaning that the fruit possesses a greater number of negative ions than positive ones. Most of the fluids that the digestive system produces (such as bile, stomach acid, and saliva) are also anionic, making lemon juice extremely compatible with your digestive system.

To benefit from lemons' natural healing properties, it's important that you use whole, fresh, organic lemons. The lemons available in a grocery store, or sometimes even a large supermarket, are usually not as "pure" as organic ones. This can be a result of overprocessing, early picking, pesticide spraying, or nutrient-depleted soils used for growing— or all the above!

Using fresh-squeezed, organic lemon juice increases the number of toxins you can eliminate each and every day you take your colon drink. (Remember the 1.87 million toxins we totaled up in Chapter 1? Are you still counting your own?) The more toxins you can flush out of your system, the more your colon will be receptive to your colon-cleansing efforts.

Why Are Oxygen-Based Colon Cleansers Used?

My professional and personal experience, as well as my extensive research on the subject, has convinced me that the most effective way to cleanse the entire intestinal tract and colon is with an oxygen-based cleanser.

This type of cleanser uses a controlled reaction to release pure, monatomic oxygen straight into the bowels. At this point you'll be

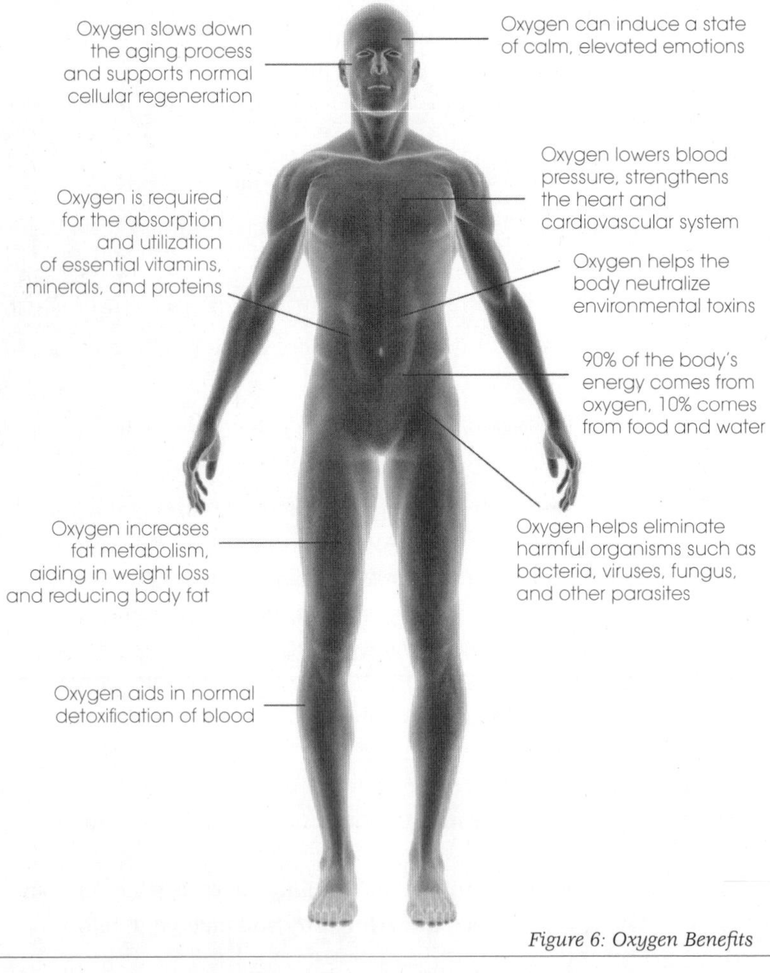

Oxygen slows down the aging process and supports normal cellular regeneration

Oxygen can induce a state of calm, elevated emotions

Oxygen is required for the absorption and utilization of essential vitamins, minerals, and proteins

Oxygen lowers blood pressure, strengthens the heart and cardiovascular system

Oxygen helps the body neutralize environmental toxins

90% of the body's energy comes from oxygen, 10% comes from food and water

Oxygen increases fat metabolism, aiding in weight loss and reducing body fat

Oxygen helps eliminate harmful organisms such as bacteria, viruses, fungus, and other parasites

Oxygen aids in normal detoxification of blood

Figure 6: Oxygen Benefits

wondering what monatomic oxygen is. Well, it may sound technical and complicated, but it's basically just a single, unbonded atom of oxygen (that is, one not attached to any other atom). The air you breathe is actually 02, or 2 oxygen molecules bonded together.

Oxygen-based cleansers use specialized forms of ozonated magnesium oxides, which are used to break down the solid toxic mass in the colon into a liquid or gas, making it easier to pass from the body in a bowel movement. In this type of cleanser, oxygen-singlet atoms are bonded to a magnesium compound. The hydrochloric acid in your stomach, or the acid in lemon juice or any other acids in your bowel, release these bonds, thus allowing monotomic oxygen to escape into the intestines.

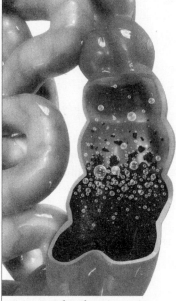

Oxygen is what's known as a "lively element." If you're using a good oxygen cleanser, it will pump enough oxygen into your bowels to literally burrow through the toxic sludge and contaminated mucus caked along the sides of your intestines. The vital oxygen in these cleansers clears out the colon, provides a great remedy for constipation, and aids in regular maintenance cleansing, too.

Not only that, but as the years of waste literally melt away and get flushed down the toilet, the intestinal lining hidden beneath it is revealed. In most cases, this lining is littered with microscopic holes caused by years of abuse or neglect. In a toxic colon, holes

Figure 7: Colon-cleansing Action

are a *bad* thing, since they can allow toxins to enter the bloodstream. After cleansing the colon, the perfect opportunity occurs for oxygen to work its way into the bloodstream where it can help restore and detoxify the entire body.

I should point out that, while I recommend that you use a good, oxygen-based intestinal cleanser, such products are not all created equal. As with any health product, it's important that you do your homework before you start experimenting with your body. Many so-called oxygen cleansers simply don't release enough oxygen to do much good.

In independent laboratory tests, only two oxygen-based cleansing products have been shown to release the amount of oxygen needed to thoroughly cleanse the intestines. Those two products are Homozon and Oxy-Powder.

Homozon has been around since the early 1900s and is considered to be the granddaddy of all oxygen cleansers. In many ways, it's a product shrouded in mystery. Its exact manufacturing processes remains a secret to this day. Debate even rages over who developed the original formula. Some say that Nicola Tesla (the famed inventor and electrical engineer) and a Dr. F. M. Eugene Blass developed the process in a hotel room in Paris. And while Homozon is an amazing product, it's not widely marketed, which makes it hard to find.

Up until this point I've avoided making any shameless plugs to promote my own personal line of health supplements. In this particular case, however, it would be wrong for me not to make an exception.

For years, I exclusively recommended Homozon to the patients who came to my clinic. Time and time again I was stunned by its effectiveness. I saw people's health make a complete turnabout— sometimes literally overnight. Even among oxygen cleansers, this one truly stood out above and beyond the other copycat products of its type.

Needless to say, I had a lot of respect for this product, and I still do. But over the years I began to notice some drawbacks and heard complaints from my patients who used it. First, the product was hard to get, and at my clinic we would often have to wait a couple months or longer before receiving a small shipment. Second, it came as a loose powder that had to be mixed with water and lemon juice, resulting in a peculiar-tasting, chalky concoction. Patients would do a "silent protest" by not taking it regularly because of its taste, or they would gag when trying to ingest it.

I knew that the world needed access to a product that was as safe and gentle as Homozon. I also knew that such a product simply had to come in an easy-to-take, vegetarian capsule so that people would use it regularly and benefit from it. So I began to look into having it made for my own practice, and perhaps for the wider world, as well.

Years later, with the help of a world-renowned oxygen biochemist, Oxy-Powder was created. By utilizing the advancements in technology made over the past hundred years, we were able to finally create a product proven to be more effective than any other oxygen-based cleanser in the world. With the addition of organic germanium-132, we had found the secret of maintaining intestinal health and oxygen delivery throughout the intestinal tract. Germanium-132 has been shown to improve the health of arteries, lower blood pressure, *help suppress some forms of cancer*, inhibit the growth of internal fungi, and enhance the body's utilization of oxygen. This is why I recommend Oxy-Powder in my ingredients for the Oxygen Colon Cleanse.

Why Is a Probiotic Recommended During the Oxygen Cleanse?

In my many years of practice, I have tried numerous probiotics. The reason I recommend Latero Flora is that I have seen the most dramatic results with this product. If you choose to use your own source of probiotics, both during your oxygen cleanse and on a regular basis, do your research and make sure you use a quality product.

Latero Flora has shown significant effectiveness in easing gastrointestinal symptoms and food sensitivities while enhancing digestive capacities. It has intriguing origins. It seems that an agriculturalist visiting a remote part of Iceland discovered rich-tasting vegetables that were being produced without chemicals. Returning to the United States, the agriculturalist conducted a series of studies that revealed the secret of the soil's growing power. The secret was a unique probiotic strain of Bacillus Laterosporus (BOD Strain), a naturally occurring bacterium.

I also recommend a probiotic called Lactobacillus Sporogenes.

Just as the planet Earth holds an abundance of life forms—some existing harmoniously, others struggling fitfully against each other—so too does the human body hold a vast, internal ecosystem consisting of literally thousands of billions of living microorganisms, all of which manage to coexist.

This internal ecosystem, referred to by many researchers as "human intestinal flora," dramatically influences, and to a certain degree even directs, every individual's personal state of health and well-being—including our physical and mental health, as well as our metabolism. More than 400 distinct species of microorganisms inhabit the various regions of the human digestive tract alone, making up nearly four pounds of every individual's total body weight.

This vast population of microorganisms far exceeds the number of tissue cells that compose the human body. When functioning properly, this vast unseen world:

- Helps guard your body against unfriendly bacteria

- Assists in maintaining the function of the digestive system

- Manages your body's vital chemical and hormonal balance

- Performs a vast number of needed tasks for supporting high energy levels and maintaining proper immune function

Transient microorganisms are extremely important to understand. These include food-borne microorganisms and soil-borne microorganisms that make their way into the human digestive tract and, depending on the characteristics of the specific organism involved, influence the overall health of the human system. *Transient microorganisms, as their name suggests, differ from resident microorganisms in that they do not take up permanent residence in the gastrointestinal tract.* Instead, they camp out, establishing small colonies for brief periods before dying off or being flushed from the intestinal system via normal digestive processes or peristaltic bowel action. However, in taking up temporary residence, they contribute to the digestive system's overall function and condition. For example, the lives of some of the more important resident microorganisms involved in human digestion and intestinal health depend on byproducts produced by the visiting transients.

Therefore, in many cases, these two very different types of microorganisms nonetheless enjoy a complex symbiotic relationship that may dramatically influence the health and well-being of your entire body. Bacillus Laterosporus (BOD Strain) is one of the most enigmatic of the transient "friendly" microorganisms found in the human gastrointestinal tract. Bacillus Laterosporus is a spore-bearing bacteria. This enables the encased spore to survive the stomach acids. Thus, the full benefit of Bacillus Laterosporus will bloom and flourish in the colon and establish colonies that will enhance your immune system and cleanse the colon of unwanted organisms such as *Candida*.

Eating Fresh Fruit

During the Oxygen Colon Cleanse is an ideal time for you to feed your body sufficient amounts of fresh organic or locally grown fruit. You will eat *only* fruit during the 6-day cleanse. Not only does fruit supply the body with the right kind of energy to draw out unwanted substances, it also ensures that the colon remains well-hydrated so that it will be an ideal environment to support the elimination and cleansing process. Fresh fruits support the elimination process by providing water, oxygen, live fiber, pectin, and vital nutrients. Also, fruits are easy to carry with you wherever you go (even in your shoulder bag or briefcase), making it easy for you to stay on the 6-day cleanse during work hours, short travel, or other daily activities.

Fruits will provide you with the energy you will need during your cleanse. In addition, they break down easily and prevent the body from expending a lot of energy. You should eat *5 times* daily during the 6-day cleanse. This might sound hard, but when you think about it, it really only takes about two minutes to peel and enjoy a banana, or eat an apple, or wash and nibble on some strawberries.

I have chosen the following fruits (listed in alphabetical order) as the best ones to assist you in the cleansing process. It's a good idea to vary the fruits throughout the day and week, both to give your system some variety and to avoid getting bored by sameness. If the fruits I recommend are not in season, or you have a hard time finding them, you can use organic apples or bananas (which are typically available year round) as a replacement.

THE OXYGEN COLON CLEANSE FRUITS

Apples	Figs	Peaches	Raspberries
Avocado	Grapefruit	Pears	Strawberries
Bananas	Mango	Persimmon	Tomatoes
Blackberries	Oranges	Pineapples	Watermelon
Blueberries	Papaya	Prunes	White grapes

EXAMPLE: Eat grapefruit for breakfast, white grapes for the midmorning snack, pineapple for lunch, oranges for the midafternoon snack, and avocados for dinner. Fruits must be eaten alone, not in combination.

NOTE: Remember to chew each bite of fruit 25 times before swallowing, or at least chew until the fruit has turned into a liquid. *Proper digestion begins in the mouth, with proper chewing.* Chewing your food will help the body absorb its vital nutrients better and more rapidly, and will also help with the cleansing process. See Chapter 5 for more details and tips on foods.

The Colon Cleanse Program

Days 1–6

ON AWAKENING

○ Make your daily colon drink. Drink 20 ounces of it (2$\frac{1}{2}$ 8-ounce glasses) from the time you make your drink to the time you eat breakfast.

○ Repeat the following Affirmation 9 times:
I AM Clean and Healthy.

BREAKFAST

○ Eat as much fruit as you can until you are full. Eat only 1 type of fruit!

- Choose one of the following: grapefruit, white grapes, watermelon, pineapple, or orange
- After breakfast and before your midmorning snack, consume another 20 ounces (2 ½ 8-ounce glasses) of the colon drink.
- Repeat the following Affirmation 9 times:
  I AM Clean and Healthy.
- Take 3 capsules of Latero Flora or other good probiotic supplement.

MIDMORNING SNACK
(HALFWAY BETWEEN BREAKFAST AND LUNCH)

- Eat as much fruit as you can until you are full. Eat only 1 type of fruit!
- Choose one of the following: blackberries, raspberries, strawberries, or blueberries. If berries are not in season, replace with apples or bananas.
- After your midmorning snack and before your lunch, consume another 20 ounces (2 ½ 8-ounce glasses) of the colon drink.
- Repeat the following Affirmation 9 times:
  I AM Clean and Healthy.

LUNCH

- Eat as much fruit as you can until you are full. Eat only 1 type of fruit!
- Choose one of the following: apple, papaya, or banana
- After lunch and before your midafternoon snack, consume another 20 ounces (2 ½ 8-ounce glasses) of the colon drink.
- Repeat the following Affirmation 9 times:
  I AM Clean and Healthy.

MIDAFTERNOON SNACK
(HALFWAY BETWEEN LUNCH AND DINNER)

- Eat as much fruit as you can until you are full. Eat only 1 type of fruit!
- Choose one of the following: grapefruit, white grapes, pineapple, or orange
- After your midafternoon snack and before your dinner, consume another 20 ounces (2 ½ 8-ounce glasses) of the colon drink.
- Repeat the following Affirmation 9 times:
  I AM Clean and Healthy.

DINNER

○ Eat as much fruit as you can until you are full. Eat only 1 type of fruit!

○ Choose one of the following: avocados or tomatoes. (Tomatoes need to be vine ripened, for best results.) You may use fresh lime juice, natural sea salt (preferably Himalayan), cayenne, or black pepper to season the avocado or tomato if necessary. It is, however, best to eat them raw.

○ After your dinner meal and before bed, consume another 20 ounces (2 ¹/₂ 8-ounce glasses) of the colon drink.

○ Repeat the following Affirmation 9 times:
  I AM Clean and Healthy.

BEFORE BED

○ Repeat the following Affirmation 9 times:
  I AM Clean and Healthy.

○ Take 6 capsules of either Oxy-Powder or a good oxygen-based cleanser with the remaining 8 ounces of the colon drink. If you do not have 3 to 5 bowel movements the following day, increase your dosage by 2 capsules each night until you achieve 3 to 5 bowel movements the following day. For the remaining days of the colon cleanse, take this same dosage every night before going to bed. After you have completed the 6-day cleanse, take your maintenance dosage as needed see below.

MAINTENANCE DOSAGE

To maintain a healthy intestinal tract, now that you have done a complete cleanse, I recommend regular cleansing at least twice per week. Use the same dosage you used for your 6-day cleanse. This amount can be taken indefinitely without its becoming habit forming or harmful to your body. Taking a regular maintenance dose of an oxygen-based colon cleanser helps supply your entire body with beneficial oxygen and aids in the natural cleansing of your intestinal tract.

Once you have completed the cleanse, I recommend following the Colon Diet, detailed in Chapter 5. After you read that chapter, you will be ready for the big task of slowly eliminating toxins from your environment. See Part 2 of this book for specific instructions.

Five Tips to Maximize the Oxygen Colon Cleanse

As you probably know, your abdomen houses many of the most vital organs in your body. The abdominal cavity houses the stomach, gallbladder, pancreas, diaphragm, colon, small intestine, and liver (collectively called the viscera). When something weakens the digestive system, such as an illness or practicing a sedentary lifestyle, the abdomen can suffer.

ABDOMINAL MASSAGE

Massage of the abdomen is a method of keeping it strong. It has been used by numerous cultures around the world for centuries as a means of promoting health. Happily, abdominal massage requires no prescription or special equipment and costs nothing but a bit of time. It has the added bonus that you can perform it on yourself, as well as on your friends, significant other, spouse, or children.

Some of the key benefits of abdominal massage are:

○ Blood flow is increased to the abdominal cavity, which in turn delivers more life-sustaining oxygen to the vital organs.

○ By stimulating internal natural processes, massage helps remove toxins.

○ Built-up fecal matter is dislodged from the walls of the intestinal tract.

○ Massage provides basic comfort and heat through touch therapy.

○ In females, massage helps realign the pelvic bone and uterus to their proper position (as they move throughout life and become misaligned).

○ Massage relieves tension and relaxes the muscles surrounding the colon, promoting a healthier digestive system.

○ Massage releases unprocessed emotional charges (that is, nervous tension).

I recommend abdominal massage highly for anyone thinking about doing a colon cleanse to detoxify their body. Practicing abdominal massage can greatly enhance the cleansing procedure by toning your colon's internal musculature for improved strength and resilience.

The following chart is a condensed set of instructions for performing an abdominal self-massage.

Your intestines may not seem to respond to your massage treatments right away, as they have likely become sluggish from years of eating bad foods and through loss of muscle tone. After practicing your technique for some time, however, you may begin to notice increased warmth from improved blood flow and a gradual lessening of tension in the abdominal area. As you attain a level of comfort and effectiveness, your massage treatments will probably require less time for the same amount of benefit.

Abdominal massage also promotes inner harmony by relaxing the body. In our hyperpaced, work-focused culture, many people walk around in a perpetual state of tension, multitasking with cell phones or electronic notepads. This habit of constant nervous anxiety isn't good for us mentally, emotionally, or physically—it can lead to the colon

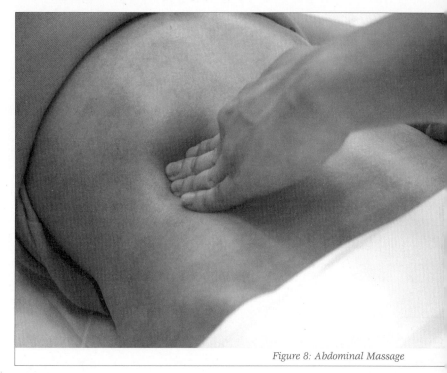

Figure 8: Abdominal Massage

becoming easily irritated by otherwise harmless stimuli whenever stress levels become elevated.

When done as a complement to a thorough colon-cleansing regimen, abdominal massage helps your body become "centered," or balanced. You'll feel better physically and emotionally after a soothing massage session. Just think about how relaxed and stress-free you feel

Abdominal Massage Technique

Characteristic Instructions and Considerations

BREATHING	Breathe in deeply and slowly—in through the nostrils and out through the mouth. This will help develop your internal breathing power, sometimes known as your chi.
LOCATION	Lying in bed or on a couch is ideal, though you may also massage while taking a warm, relaxing bath or reclined on a lounge chair in the early morning or late afternoon sun. Try to lie as flat as possible.
HAND PLACEMENT	Begin with your hands just above the groin area on your lower abdomen. You can elevate your upper arms with small pillows to extend your reach and allow the hands a beneficial vantage point for pushing down. Work upward to include the entire abdomen.
PRESSURE	Always apply light pressure and avoid compressing painful areas. Use your entire hand, and coordinate your technique with natural breathing so that you are not pushing down as your abdomen is expanding. While it takes practice to develop your own sense of "touch" for massage, you should try to maintain constancy in the pressure used. Focus on feeling the softness of your intestines beneath the skin, on natural contractions and movement, on blockages that diminish or go away, and on improved "flow" within your entire digestive system.
RHYTHM	Your hands lift lightly as you're breathing in, and they push downward with mild to medium pressure as you're breathing out.
TECHNIQUE	Use small circular motions, alternating clockwise and counterclockwise, with the left hand on the left side of the abdomen and the right hand on the right side of the abdomen. Work hands toward each other and then away. Experiment with different patterns such as elongated ovals, zigzags, and small "rubbing" strokes. You can also vary which parts of your hands apply the pressure. Determine through experience which movements benefit you most.
TIME	Self-massage sessions should last between 15 and 30 minutes, with a 5-minute "warm-up" phase to develop your rhythm and force, and, as your massage ends, a 5-minute "cool-down" phase to gradually ease the pressure applied.
VISUALIZATION	Water imagery is especially beneficial, as water is constantly flowing, never occupying the same space twice, changing with each new wave to create a beautiful, unique expression of nature. The human body, mind, and spirit all resonate with the liquid formlessness of water. Imagine rising and drifting weightlessly on a vast, calm ocean while performing the massage.

after receiving a deep-tissue back massage. You can receive the same benefits from massaging your abdomen, as well. In all of your health-related exercises, keep in mind that a clean, healthy colon is one of the strongest assets you can have for preventing illness and disease.

DAILY BREATHING

Practicing simple breathing exercises—such as slow, diaphragmatic breathing and conscious muscle relaxation—can help you clear your mind and calm your physical responses to stress. By relieving daily stress you also relax your bowels. In addition, deep, focused breathing increases the blood's oxygen content. Organs such as the colon depend on sufficient amounts of oxygen.

The technique: Breathe in deeply through your nose for 4 seconds. Hold your breath for 16 seconds, and then release the air through your mouth gradually over 8 seconds. Repeat this exercise 9 times to complete a session. Try to do at least 2 sessions daily, or whenever you feel stressed.

FOCUS ON POSITIVE EMOTIONS

It's easy to get wrapped up in today's busy world, and to focus more on the negative instead of the positive (what's "wrong" with a colleague or a family member, rather than what's "right" with them). Negative stressors surround us, but we shouldn't let ourselves be overwhelmed by them. If you're feeling stressed, anxious, angry, or depressed, whatever the cause might be, there's a good chance that your colon is aware of it. Think of how your stomach instantly tightens when something shocking or surprising happens. Stressful situations and emotions release hormones in the body that can have detrimental effects on our digestive health.

To avoid such effects, surround yourself with positive energy. This could take many forms. Listen to your favorite music, get a massage, take a walk with a friend, brush and play with your pet, and don't forget to *smile*; smiling is contagious, and can only positively affect the people around you. If you're having a hard time dealing with negative emotions, find someone to talk to, whether it's a close nonjudgmental friend, a spiritual counselor, or a professional therapist.

Stress relief, I believe, is critical for optimal health. A chronically tense state of mind will not help detoxify the colon—it will only contribute to its toxicity. So please do whatever it takes to decrease the negative energy forces in your life, and replace them with stress-reducing, positive energy forces. Live in the *now*.

GET PLENTY OF SLEEP

It's really hard for a lot of people to get sufficient sleep. Somehow, Americans manage to overdo things and underdo others. We typically overdo things when we're in stressful environments such as at our workplace, and we underdo things in life-sustaining activities such as exercise, healthy eating, rest, and sleep. Working too hard and not getting enough sleep is completely the reverse of what nature intends for us. Sleep is one of the most essential activities that we perform. Good sleep is not a recommendation or suggestion—it's a requirement. The body absolutely has to have time to rest and recuperate.

It's important to retire to bed early (at 8 to 9 p.m., or by 10 p.m. at the latest) in order to receive the beneficial, regenerative magnetic fields of the earth. Sleeping for two to five hours before midnight enables our bodies to increase the natural healing powers of our immune system that are necessary in restoring health. It also aids the morning elimination cycle. Try to sleep in the darkest environment possible. When light hits the eyes, it disrupts the sleep rhythm of the pineal gland and the production of beneficial hormones such as melatonin and serotonin.

GET REGULAR CHIROPRACTIC ADJUSTMENTS

The human body is an intricate mechanism made up of millions of nerves that execute our every move. One such impressive group of nerves is located in the lumbar (lowest) region of the spine. The nerves there are responsible for controlling our body's bowel, urinary, and sexual functions. When these nerves become either overactive or underactive, whether from a cause such as a herniated or bulging disc, a pinched nerve, or even a slight misalignment of the vertebrae, all three of these important functions can suffer.

The lumbar nerves control intestinal peristalsis, the wave-like contractions that help move waste through the body. Sometimes, pressure on these nerves can limit peristalsis and thus allow an onset of constipation or diarrhea. When these nerves are affected, you may feel some pain or discomfort that spreads across your abdomen, experience nausea, or even temporarily lose control of your bowels.

Sometimes having a chiropractor do a simple spinal realignment is all that's needed to relieve pressure on the nerves. Incorporating a routine chiropractic exam and spinal alignment into your health regimen can help keep this important group of nerves from being compromised. Your chiropractor can also demonstrate some exercises to add to your routine that will strengthen and support the lumbar area of the spine to help prevent these types of problems in the future.

Questions and Answers on the Oxygen Colon Cleanse

Q. Can I do this cleanse and still carry on my daily activities?

A. Yes, you can keep on with your regular routine while doing the cleanse. Just mix your gallon of ingredients and take it with you if you'll be away from home. For food, also take your fresh fruit with you (you can clean and cut it up at home and put into a sealed container).

Tip: It's best to start a 6-day cleanse on a Friday or Saturday morning; that timing will give you greater access to a bathroom for longer periods, might relax you a bit, and will also let your body become accustomed to cleanse-related changes over the weekend. Continuing the 6-day cleanse should be manageable so long as you have a bathroom nearby.

Q. Am I going to be stuck in the bathroom all day long?

A. For the first few days, depending on your weight, you may need to stay close to a bathroom. Yet some people who have a lot of compacted fecal matter may not have a bowel movement until the second or third day. Each person's results will be different. After all, you probably spent years (if not decades) slowly building up the toxic waste in your digestive system, so naturally it may take a little time to break down. The average number of bowel movements daily during the cleanse is 3 to 7.

Q. Will I lose weight during the 6 days of cleansing?

A. This cleanse is not specifically intended for weight loss. While some people have reported weight loss ranging from 5 to 20 pounds when cleansing, this is not actual fat loss, but rather is due to the elimination of stored, hard-compacted fecal matter throughout the entire length of the intestinal tract.

Q. How will I know when my bowels are clean and the old compacted fecal matter is gone?

A. Everyone's results on the cleanse will differ, depending on their diet, exercise patterns, and age, as well as physical and emotional stress levels. However, to ensure that you continue to stay as clean inside as possible, you should eat only live, raw fruits and vegetables and should completely eliminate as many environmental toxins as possible (see Part 2). Because the Standard American Diet (appropriately called

"SAD") is so poor, you will need to cleanse on a continuous basis to help keep the entire intestinal lining clean. Therefore, I recommend a continued maintenance dose using a oxygen based cleanser 2 to 3 times weekly (especially after the consumption of red meat meals). Use your bowel activity as a guide. You will know how "clean" you are by the color, consistency, and frequency of your bowel movements. As your intestinal tract becomes progressively cleaner, the color of each succeeding bowel movement should be much lighter, and transit time (time from eating to elimination) should be shorter (12 to 16 hours). You should also be experiencing more frequent, softer, and smoother bowel movements. See Chapter 3 for details on normal stool evaluation.

Q. How often should I repeat the Oxygen Cleanse?

A. Feel free to repeat the Oxygen Cleanse to suit your needs. Factors will include what your typical diet consists of, the amount of toxins you expose yourself to daily, stressors in your life, and how well you feel generally. I recommend that you repeat the 6-day cleanse every 3 to 6 months if any of the following three conditions apply:

○ Your diet regularly includes processed or fast foods, coffee, soft drinks, or alcohol.

○ You're experiencing constipation or you feel compacted.

○ You do not exercise regularly (that is, 3 times per week or more often).

○ You experience regular yeast infections, bloating or gas.

Even if you follow my suggestions and eliminate toxins (as best you can) in your environment, improve your diet, and ramp up your exercise routine, you should still repeat the 6-day cleanse every 6 months, to help maintain optimal intestinal health.

TIP: To check the time it takes for food to go through your system (its "transit time"), consume an entire ear of corn one evening with dinner. Chart the time of the dinner meal. Do not eat any corn 3 days prior to testing. Then, watch for the corn to appear in your stool. As soon as you see the kernels in the stool, chart the day and time. This will be your current transit time. For accuracy I recommend repeating the corn test 2 or 3 times.

Q. What makes the Oxygen Colon Cleanse so different from other colon cleansing programs?

A. The Oxygen Colon Cleanse is distinctly better than others primarily in its ability to clean the entire 25- to 30-foot length of the digestive tract. It's designed to clean it thoroughly and to oxidize it, and reduce the amount of hard, impacted fecal matter in the small and large intestines and the colon. This cleanse uses oxygen O^2 from the fruit and monotomic oxygen O^1 in the cleanser) to release useful oxygen into the bloodstream and bowel, and does so in a natural, nontoxic way. Estimates predict the average person by the age of 40 has between 10 to 20 pounds of hard, compacted fecal matter lodged in their intestinal tract. Since the human intestinal tract is 25 to 30 feet long, if you were to cut it open and spread it out (horrible thought), the surface area would be the size of a tennis court. By using this cleanse you can melt away or oxidize the compaction from the small intestine, the large intestine, and the colon—safely and effectively. This is critical to do, because, as you know full well by now, a clean intestinal tract is an essential step in achieving optimal health.

Q. What symptoms might I experience during the 6-day cleanse?

A. During a cleanse you may experience watery or gaseous stools, noisy bowel sounds, or some temporary cramping caused by gas buildup. Cramping should subside after 2 or 3 days. Other temporary effects may include low grade headaches or joint or muscle pain, draining sinuses, fatigue, skin eruptions, and insomnia. All of them will resolve as soon as the toxins are expelled from the body.

The Overnight "Quick Colon Cleanse"

Let's say you go out for dinner and overeat and possibly overdrink. Eating too much at the dinner meal can wreak havoc on the colon, let alone on how you will feel the next day. The steak, potatoes, wine, dessert, and everything else you consumed can sit in your intestinal tract for two to three days, because the improper mixing of foods causes the steak to putrefy, the carbohydrates to ferment, and the fats to turn rancid before they can be processed and then eliminated. Such an overload of food also depletes the enzymes needed to properly break the food down. In addition, most people are so eager to binge at a party meal they do not chew their food properly, thereby causing bigger chunks of food to move into the GI tract.

I am not recommending that you eat and drink like this on a regular basis. Yet with our culture being the way it is, and the poor quality of restaurant food being the way it is, you may find it difficult to avoid an occasional dinner party where you eat too much, or a night of indulgence at home.

But if you do decide to splurge once in a while, it is better to get that garbage out of your system as soon as possible. An overnight "quick cleanse" is the easiest and fastest way.

Technique: Before bed, squeeze the juice of 1/4 lemon (preferably organic) and add 1 teaspoon of organic apple cider vinegar into 16 ounces of purified water or distilled water, and drink it along with 8 capsules of Oxy-Powder or other high-quality, oxygen-based cleanser.

Note: Because your stomach is full and therefore probably distended, you might experience some cramping after you consume all your drink. If that happens, get up and walk around for 15 minutes or so, to increase blood flow and let gravity pull the food down. The next day, everything should be eliminated safely and effectively.

Can I Use Any Other Colon Cleansing Methods?

In the wide spectrum of colon cleansing, options include colon hydrotherapy, laxatives, enemas, bentonite or other cleansing clays, herbal supplements, and oxygen-based cleansers. Colon hydrotherapy and enemas are both mechanical methods of cleansing that involve the use of specialized equipment. Laxatives and natural supplements, including oxygen-based cleansers (discussed earlier), are usually administered orally or rectally.

It's important that you become as well informed as possible before you choose *any* method to cleanse your colon. The sections below cover all essential aspects of the major colon-cleansing options, including their advantages as well as their drawbacks.

As you know, colon cleansing methods are designed to remove the toxic waste that pollutes your intestines. You also know that constipation is often one of the first signs of toxic buildup, and that clearing out all that toxic buildup with regular cleansing can and get

---

TIP: Alcohol drinkers who use the Overnight "Quick Colon Cleanse" report having reduced hangover symptoms the next day and often have a renewed sense of energy.

things flowing. Constipation treatment, however, may not necessarily involve colon cleansing, especially if the problem is addressed according to traditional medical guidelines. Basically, a good intestinal cleanser will attack the source of the constipation, while traditional constipation treatments, such as laxatives, may only temporarily relieve constipation symptoms and may do little or nothing to address the compaction or the healing of the delicate intestinal tissue.

Can Laxatives Cleanse My Colon?

Around $850 million is spent every year on laxatives in the United States. They are usually the first thing that comes to mind when most people think about relieving constipation. Yet laxatives carry some serious risks, and in no way are they a true cleansing solution.

Laxatives come in many different types. They use various methods to achieve the same results—eliminating intestinal blockage. Generally speaking, they can be lumped into three categories: osmotic laxatives, stimulant laxatives, and bulk-forming laxatives.

OSMOTIC LAXATIVES cause excess fluids to be drawn into the intestines, by osmosis. This is a slow process that can take up to several days, but eventually it increases the stool's fluid bulk, basically turning it into diarrhea so that it's easier to pass. This type of laxative can also cause severe dehydration due to water loss, as well as cramping and bloating due to gas buildup during the initial waiting period.

Osmotic laxatives include lactulose (Duphalac, Generlac, Actilax), sorbitol, glycerin (Colace), polyethylene glycol compounds (Mira LAX), and magnesium hydroxide (milk of magnesia).

STIMULANT LAXATIVES are made with harsh, often toxic, chemicals that cause the intestinal muscles to spasm and contract. Their popularity stems from the fact that they can begin to work in a matter of hours. Unfortunately, they can also cause the same diarrhea, dehydration, and gas-related pain as osmotic laxatives. And, if overused, stimulant laxatives can become incredibly addictive and even cause long-term damage to the sensitive intestinal lining. The intestines can quickly grow dependent on them to trigger a "false" bowel movement, thus preventing normal intestinal contractions. This condition, known as "lazy bowel syndrome," ultimately results in a long-term battle with chronic constipation and the loss of muscle tone and strength surrounding the bowel, as well as embarrassing accidents on occasion.

Stimulant laxatives include senna, cascara sagrada, castor oil, Dulcolax, Ex-Lax Gentle Nature, Fleet Bisacodyl, Gentlax, and Senokot.

BULK-FORMING LAXATIVES use highly absorbent materials (typically dead fiber rather than live fiber, such as a fresh apple) to increase the overall mass of the stool in the bowel. As the stool increases in size, the bowels are forced to expend excess energy and work harder to expel clogged fecal matter.

Fiber and increased stool mass are both usually good things. But bulk-forming laxatives can be dangerous, since they have the potential to clog the bowels. This may be due to the ingredient psyllium, which is used in most over-the-counter fiber laxatives such as Metamucil. Psyllium is one of the most common herbal ingredients used in colon cleansers, and especially in over-the-counter fiber laxatives.

Numerous reports have been received of serious allergic reactions following the ingestion of psyllium products. These reactions include labored breathing, skin irritations or hives, and potentially life-threatening anaphylaxis. Long-term use of products containing psyllium may also negatively affect absorption of certain essential vitamins and minerals, including iron. Perhaps most ironically, obstruction of the gastrointestinal tract has also been regularly cited in studies of patients taking psyllium products improperly (not having read and followed the instructions on the label, and often not drinking enough water). These studies seem to suggest that this problem is especially common in individuals who are prone to suffering from constipation.

Other potentially harmful fiber laxatives include methylcellulose (Citrucel), calcium polycarbophil (FiberCon), and wheat dextrin (Benefiber).

What Herbal Colon-Cleansing Ingredients Should I Be Aware Of?

The natural health-supplement industry has recently been flooded with numerous "infomercials" on natural health, herbal colon cleansers, and detoxifiers. These may be natural, but virtually none of them is effective at ridding the colon of toxins.. According to the National Library of Medicine, the National Institutes of Health, and similar organizations, many herbal colon cleansers not only could be ineffective but also could put consumer health at serious risk.

Most manufacturers choose to include cheap and potentially dangerous ingredients in their formulations. Popular herbal ingredients to be especially wary of include psyllium, cascara sagrada, and senna.

Many other potentially dangerous herbal combinations make their way into herbal cleansers, so be sure to research each and every individual ingredient in *any* herbal cleanser before putting it into your body.

Psyllium is a bulk-forming laxative that's high in both fiber and mucilage. The laxative properties of psyllium (which is the seed of the fleawort plant, an Old World plantain) are due to the swelling of the husk when it comes in contact with water. When ingested, the resulting bulk stimulates a reflex contraction of the walls of the bowel. The psyllium acts as a hard sponge as it works its way down. This often causes an emptying of the bowel.

While psyllium may be marketed for short-term bowel emptying, it is not effective in fully cleansing the bowel, removing much of the toxic waste, or improving the long-term health of the intestinal walls.

Despite the claims of many manufacturers, use of laxatives or constipation relievers containing psyllium (or its components or extracts), or ingestion of this "natural" herbal supplement, can be a potentially fatal decision. A recent search on *www.shopping.com* using the keyword "psyllium" revealed over 800 products and variants containing this ingredient.

Although most psyllium-containing products offer direct-to-consumer sales, many can be found on the shelves of your neighborhood grocery store or pharmaceutical outlet under brand names. Psyllium has even been included in breakfast cereal marketed at reducing cholesterol by being "heart healthy." After all (or so the consumer is meant to think), if it's included in breakfast cereal, there can't be anything unsafe about it—right?

These products' manufacturers must be aware of the risk of using psyllium, as they include warnings on the labels similar to the ones below (chosen randomly).

PSYLLIUM WARNINGS

○ "Taking this product without adequate fluid may cause it to swell and block your throat or esophagus and may cause choking."

○ "Do not take this product if you have difficulty in swallowing."

○ "If you experience chest pain, vomiting, or difficulty in swallowing or breathing after taking this product, seek immediate medical attention."

○ "Keep out of reach of children."

○ "In case of overdose, get medical help or contact a Poison Control Center right away."

○ "*Allergy Alert:* This product may cause an allergic reaction in people sensitive to inhaled or ingested psyllium.

Ask a doctor before use if you have:

> ○ A sudden change in bowel habits persisting for 2 weeks
>
> ○ Abdominal pain, nausea, or vomiting

○ Stop use and ask a doctor if: Constipation lasts more than 7 days or rectal bleeding occurs. These may be signs of a serious condition."

Senna, an herb, is a stimulant laxative that is toxic to animal muscle tissue, yet this substance is a common ingredient added every day in the manufacture of herbal teas, weight-loss supplements, vitamins, and especially laxatives—in fact, senna is often prescribed as a "natural" medicine for curing constipation. Despite the alarming fact of its toxicity, senna continues to be included in hundreds of products while simultaneously causing a host of serious health conditions, diseases, and even death in high enough amounts.

When senna becomes highly concentrated in the organs or bloodstream, through overconsumption by whatever means, this herb can lead to the recipient's developing a variety of detrimental health concerns. Senna seems to affect primarily body systems related to the blood or natural cellular functions, or both, but it can also severely damage the liver. Common diseases and conditions caused by senna overuse or toxicity include:

> ○ Decreased enzyme production
>
> ○ Blood diseases
>
> ○ Liver failure
>
> ○ Musculoskeletal tissue damage
>
> ○ Nervous system impairment
>
> ○ Decreased energy production
>
> ○ Unhealthy weight loss
>
> ○ Severe diarrhea
>
> ○ Diaper rash and blisters (in infants and toddlers)
>
> ○ Death of colorectal tissue *(possibly leading to colon cancer)*

Cascara sagrada is also a stimulant laxative that has been demonstrated, through scientific processes, to actually cause serious digestive problems, including worsening symptoms such as diarrhea and constipation rather than relieving them. Other health conditions you can develop by using cascara sagrada include:

- Acute hepatitis (swelling of the liver)
- Liver damage
- Abdominal pain
- Rectal bleeding
- Lesions in the colon

Cascara is one of a group of herbal plants classified as anthraquinones—known cancer-causing agents. In other words, when lab animals are introduced to this herb in sufficient quantities, tumors or colon cancer often result. Only a fractional amount of DNA differentiates human beings from many other mammals, such as rats, primates, or even a household fly...so whatever can kill one animal can probably kill *most* animals.

You obviously don't want to ingest this herb or any of its derivatives. Take the time to seek out a product supporting your body's ability to cleanse and heal itself, rather than forcing a dangerous laxative effect to occur that can cause more harm than good.

One popular but disreputable tactic used by companies selling herbal cleansers is to show pictures of reported "mucoid plaque ropes" deposited in the toilet. Don't let these disgusting strands of half-digested fiber fool you—there is no proof that these "mucoid ropes" are the built-up toxic matter actually being excreted. I have created this same mucoid substance in the lab by mixing psyllium with some white flour, some hydrogenated oil, and water. You end up with a foul-looking but easily molded paste.

These products can be fairly inexpensive ($20 or so for a month's supply) or can be outrageously priced (about $100 for a month's supply). They usually require multiple steps, mixing different bags of ingredients, followed by a set regimen, and can be time consuming and messy. I myself would rather take a couple of pills before I go to bed at night.

These days, many people pursuing better intestinal health state that they have benefited from bulk-forming colon cleansers. My attitude is that if it makes them feel better, great! I am not one to say that what works for one person doesn't necessarily work for others. But I do stress that it's up to you to make an educated decision for your own health. I'm not cautioning you not to use these if nothing else is available—simply urging you to use caution and see what works best for you.

Are Enemas Effective at Cleansing the Colon?

Enemas are one of the oldest-known techniques for cleansing the colon and treating constipation. People all over the world have used them for centuries.

In its simplest form, an enema is a device that is inserted into the anus in order to inject fluid (historically, just water) from a holding bag into the rectum. This can be an effective method for removing waste that has become trapped in the lowest part of the colon, but it does little to actually cleanse the full intestinal tract.

Besides plain water, a number of different solutions have been used in enemas. Herbal blends, oils, coffee, and diluted clay are only a few of the more popular examples.

There are even so-called "dry enemas" that achieve a similar effect by injecting small amounts of sterile lubricant, such as nonmedicated glycerin, directly into the rectum using a disposable, nonhypodermic syringe. This works much like a suppository, but it produces an effect much more quickly. Some people prefer dry enemas to their wet counterparts simply because they aren't as messy. Less fluid going into the bowels, in their view, means less fluid coming out afterward.

Enemas can be genuinely useful for occasionally treating an acute case of constipation. Their effectiveness, though, is somewhat limited and depends largely on the type of solution used in them. Also, because they are only able to efficiently loosen waste sitting at the *end* of the bowels, they aren't a good long-term solution for preventing constipation or removing upper-intestinal toxins.

Many people are also understandably uneasy about the idea of inserting something into their anus. Another thing to keep in mind is that enemas can be more than merely a little uncomfortable—if administered incorrectly, they can cause serious damage to delicate tissues.

DOCTOR'S NOTE: In my practice I have used enemas consisting of organic coffee, organic herbals, and organic clay with great success, depending on the condition I was treating as well as the toxicity and health concerns of the patient. Talk to your natural health care provider to see whether you can benefit from these particular types of enemas.

Bentonite Clay

One particular kind of clay, bentonite, has been heralded for its internal cleansing properties. This all-natural clay has been used to help individuals afflicted with several symptoms of constipation (such as bloating and gas) as well as irritable bowel syndrome. As a result, bentonite clay has become a staple of many detoxification programs. When taken internally, bentonite clay provides multiple benefits, including:

- Detoxifying the liver
- Cleansing toxins from the colon
- Promoting a healthful bacterial balance in the digestive system
- Removing heavy metals and chemicals after radiation treatments
- Boosting the immune system
- Supporting efficient cellular respiration
- Improving the digestive system's assimilation of nutrients

This unique clay has powerful *adsorptive* and *absorptive* properties. While the words may sound similar, they involve completely different processes.

In *adsorption*, the molecules comprising bentonite clay are negatively charged. The molecules of toxins, harmful bacteria, and other disease-causing agents are positively charged. As the clay traverses the colon, the negative ions attract the toxic, positive ions and bond to them. Ions on the outer edges of both molecules swap sides, causing an exchange reaction that electrically "satisfies" the molecules. The two molecules are thus bound together until the clay molecule literally absorbs the toxic molecule.

In *absorption*, bentonite clay of sufficiently high quality possesses a molecular structure of only 17 minerals. Chemically speaking, the fewer minerals found in a molecule, the higher its potential of absorption of other substances. The clay acts as a sponge as it absorbs the molecules that were initially "swapped" and bonded in the adsorption process. The clay molecule takes the toxin molecule bonded to its exterior and assimilates it internally. Your body can then expel the toxin-filled clay molecules via normal bowel movements.

A word of caution: Bentonite clay should not be taken if you are pregnant, are of advanced age, or have waited less than two hours after taking any medications or nutritional supplements. No known side effects are associated with ingesting pure, organic samples of this healing clay in the recommended amounts. Still, bentonite clay has not been subject to a longitudinal study focusing on its physiological effects in humans. It's always best to consult a qualified health care practitioner before taking any new supplement. Plus, you should take the time to conduct your own research and find a supplement with a history of safety as well as high standards of purity and effectiveness.

Colon Hydrotherapy for Colon Cleansing

In a number of ways, colon hydrotherapy, also called colonic irrigation, is like a supercharged enema. Although do-it-yourself kits are available for the adventurous, I recommend having this treatment administered by a properly trained, certified, or licensed professional at a private office, clinic, or spa. Most therapists are trained to massage the abdomen gently during the release cycle. This helps move the gas and waste that is blocked in the colon. It is wise to find a therapist who uses an FDA-cleared device and also uses disposable speculums and tubing (for sanitation).

CAUTION: Colon hydrotherapy may not be suitable for people suffering from severe hemorrhoids, malignant polyps, active inflammatory bowel disease, or active diverticulitis.

The closed system is best, to prevent release of wastes back into the local municipal water supply.

It is important to be cleared for any possible risks before having this kind of treatment, especially if a woman believes she may

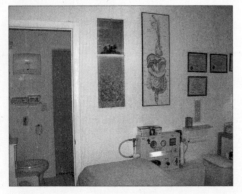

be pregnant.

During a colon hydrotherapy session, a therapist will help you, the client, gently insert a small plastic tube, called a speculum, a few inches into your rectum. The speculum is attached to a plastic hose that connects to a colon hydrotherapy device. Then warm, purified water enters your body and will slowly and gently begin to cleanse the colon. Depending on your symptoms and condition, your therapist may choose to add herbs, ozone, or enzymes to the water to increase the benefits of the therapy.

As the water flows into your colon, it causes the muscles to contract and expand, encouraging the body to expel any undigested food, water, and bacteria, as well as any gas and mucus that have built up in the colon. This compacted toxic matter leaves your body by traveling through a separate evacuation tube that leads back to the device. Warm water flows gently in and out of the colon a few times in a typical session, which lasts between 30 and 50 minutes, depending on how you feel. The treatment process is painless, and you may feel some warmth as the toxins move out of your body.

Colon hydrotherapy is extremely effective at toxin removal, especially when supplemented with the use of an oxygen-based cleanser. To maximize results, many colon hydrotherapists now use oxygen cleansers in conjunction with their regular colon hydrotherapy sessions to clean the entire intestinal tract.

> **REMINDER:** Some colon-cleansing methods can strip beneficial bacteria from the intestinal tract as they remove toxic waste. It's important, therefore, to take a probiotic supplement during any cleansing process, to ensure that the colon maintains a healthy population of beneficial bacteria. Ask your practitioner which probiotic is best for you. For me, Bacillus Laterosporus or Bacillus Sporogenes seems to work the best.

SUCCESS STORY #1

"As a child, I only had only one bowel movement per week. Therefore, I have struggled with constipation since childhood. In the beginning I went to medical doctors, but to no avail. In my twenties I still couldn't even go to the bathroom [without] taking 8 prescription pills per night. When I was 32, I was introduced by my chiropractor to healthy alternatives. I am eternally grateful for this. I am now 45 and have come a long way since then.

"From first-hand experience, I feel that combining an oxygen-based cleanser with colonics has excellent results. My goal and my healthcare professionals' goal is for me to only have to do a colonic 2 times a year. I am to the point of only needing 1 colonic per month, and I am close to being able to do 1 colonic every other month. I gauge this with being able to have more than 1 movement per day—which is a miracle of God, from where I started. In the past 2 months, I have had 2 or more movements per day! God bless you and thank you for caring!"

—*Juli B., Broken Arrow, Oklahoma*

SUCCESS STORY #2

"I was inspired to enter this field [of colon hydrotherapy] about 30 years ago when I was so sick with *Candida*/yeast overgrowth that I couldn't see to drive a car. My headaches were chronic and no painkillers were helping. I was blessed to be led to a wonderful chiropractor that had a colon hydrotherapist in his office. I began with a series of 12 sessions over the course of 6 weeks. After the first session, my vision cleared. Two weeks later my headaches disappeared, never to return. Needless to say, I was reborn in health!

"Within the next few years, I left my real estate career behind to begin practicing Colon Hydrotherapy in 1992. I now teach at our International School for Colon Hydrotherapy, Inc., in Florida. Our graduates hail from over 11 different countries and we are proud of each one of them. They share our vision to help end the suffering and assist people in finding ways toward better health. Dr. Group's Oxy-Powder is an integral part of our success. We suggest it to all of our people and we see amazing results!"

—*Cathy Shea, President, International School for Colon Hydrotherapy, Inc.*

At this point, you've probably gathered that I support colon hydrotherapy and oxygen-based cleansers the majority of the time. I do, however, also recommend bentonite clay or enemas on occasion.

Many other colon-cleansing herbs and methods are widely available. I have explained the most common methods earlier in this chapter. To put your knowledge into practice, I recommend that you spend a good deal of time carefully going over the material in Part 2 of this book. Then you can use your growing understanding of both colon cleansing and toxin exposure to pursue your goal of better health.

Is There Anything Else I Can Do to Help Keep My Colon Healthy?

You may find this surprising, but the position your body takes on the toilet can actually affect the condition and health of your bowel. Sitting on a regular toilet seat is completely unnatural, as it constricts the anal canal, resulting in incomplete evacuations. Think about it—very young children will instinctively squat to move their bowels. This is by far

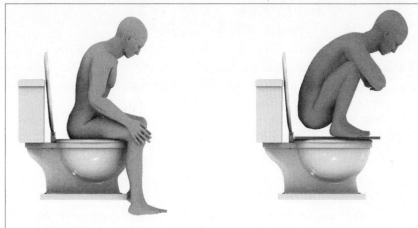

Figure 9: Awkward Sitting Position — Relaxed Squatting Position

the healthiest position to adopt if you want to prevent constipation and maintain healthy intestinal function.

USE A SQUATTING PLATFORM

I recommend using a squatting platform to encourage relaxed and complete evacuation. It may take a little getting used to, but you'll be happy you took the time to find your natural elimination position. A common platform is shown below; many varieties are available, so make sure that you find one that you'll be comfortable with and that fits your toilet design.

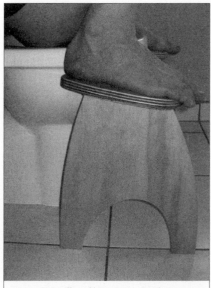

Figure 10: Lillipad Squatting Stool

For more information on these squatting stools, see the Resources section.

The cleansing methods I have shared with you till this point are not the only way to purge harmful toxins from the body and stimulate normal bowel evacuation.

The human body actually has five natural elimination routes (only four in men). These are basically paths that lead harmful poisons out of the body:

○ Defecation (bowel movements)

○ Urination (passing water)

○ Diaphoresis (sweating)

○ Respiration (breathing)

○ Menstruation (monthly bleeding in women)

All five routes can effectively purge the body of toxins, provided that the body is at peak performance.

Opening up all these elimination routes can help take some of the burden off the colon. Therefore, it's important to have all the elimination routes in good working condition. This means you have to use them consistently and efficiently.

EXERCISE TO REDUCE TOXIC BUILDUP

Exercise is the fastest and most effective way to open up the elimination routes.

Exercise can help reduce the toxic buildup in your colon, provide you with more energy, tone up your colon muscles, and neutralize toxins more efficiently—plus it will make you feel unstoppable in no time. Appropriate, regular exercise is a huge part of maintaining overall health. It can also drastically reduce your chances of developing serious diseases, such as colorectal cancer.

Remember, exercise shouldn't overexert your body. Quite as important, it should be fun. You're more likely to stick with an exercise activity if you find one or more that you really enjoy, and vary them as you wish so that you don't get bored with the same old drill three or four times a week.

Some Great Ways to Get Exercise

○ Rebounding (mini trampoline)—this is my personal favorite

○ Long, leisurely bike rides

○ Lively walking

○ Hiking

○ Swimming

○ Martial arts

○ Light jump-roping

○ Rowing

○ Pilates

○ Yoga

If it's impossible for you to set aside time for regular exercise, try to work it into your daily activities. Park in a space far away from the store entrance or your company building, take the stairs instead of the elevator, or ride your bike to work (if possible). The important thing is that you adopt an *active* lifestyle.

Trampoline Rebounding

Rebounding is an easy and fun exercise that is excellent for opening up all the elimination routes consistently and effectively. It's basically just jumping on a mini-trampoline in a controlled but fun way. It's low-impact (so it won't damage any joints), it's aerobic (that is, with oxygen—earlier we talked about how important oxygen is to the body), and it even has the seal of approval from NASA and its high-flying astronauts as being the most efficient workout ever. If you think exercise is boring, tedious, or uncomfortable, you simply have to try rebounding. Once you start bouncing, 20 or 30 minutes will have passed pleasurably (and beneficially) before you know it.

Health Benefits of Rebounding

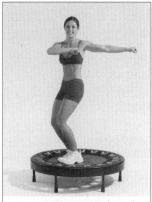

Figure 11: Rebounding

- Opens up and supports all elimination routes
- Improves circulation of oxygen to organs, including the colon
- Increases heart and lung functionality
- Strengthens the immune system
- Strengthens and drains the lymphatic system
- Boosts energy levels
- Lowers cholesterol
- Aids in digestion and massages the bowel
- Enhances metabolism
- May slow the aging process
- Reduces stress and anxiety

In addition to rebounding, the chart on page 72 will help you identify ways to maximize the amount of toxins removed from your body.

Simply put, regular intestinal cleansing eliminates toxic debris and years of compacted waste. Not only can it help reduce the symptoms and severity of a wide range of health issues, it can downright prevent

ELIMINATION ROUTE	IDEAS FOR OPENING UP ELIMINATION ROUTE
RESPIRATION (Rapid breathing from exercise) (Deep breathing)	• Participate in aerobic activity for 30 minutes a day. • Perform daily deep-breathing exercises.
DIAPHORESIS (Sweating)	• Participate in aerobic or anaerobic activity for 30 minutes a day. • Drink plenty of purified water. • Treat yourself to a far infrared or steam sauna.
DEFECATION (Bowel movement)	• Have 2 to 4 bowel movements daily. • Drink plenty of pure water. • Eat only fresh organic fruits for breakfast each morning. • Combine colon hydrotherapy with oxygen-based cleansers. • Use a squatting stool with your toilet to encourage proper waste elimination. • Don't delay when you have the urge to go.
URINATION (Passing water)	• Drink plenty of water. • Don't delay urination when you have the urge to go. • If you wake up at night to urinate, it means this elimination route is partially blocked and you need a liver, gallbladder, intestinal, heavy metal, and parasite cleanse.
MENSES (Monthly discharge in women)	• Drink plenty of water. • Avoid birth control pills, because they automatically block the elimination of toxins through menses. • Massage the lower pelvic area during menses.

them. And I'm not just talking about digestive illnesses—I mean that it can prevent disease throughout the entire human body.

Are you getting excited about cleansing your colon and opening up those elimination routes? You should be! The time has come—don't you agree?—for you to regain the health of your colon and enhance your living. But there's more to colon health than the occasional cleanse. You have to be good to your colon each and every day. In the next chapter, you'll find the best types of foods, food-type balance, and optimal meal plan to keep your colon healthy.

CHAPTER 5

The Colon Diet

You're finally on your way to achieving optimal colon health. I hope you plan to combine the benefits of colon hydrotherapy *and* oxygen colon cleansing to detoxify your colon—I highly recommend

> "The doctor of the future will give no medicine, but will interest his patients in the care of the human frame, in diet and in the cause and prevention of disease."
>
> —*Thomas A. Edison*

this one-two punch. Still, as with many things in life, there's *no quick fix*. Merely cleansing the toxins from your colon once in a while will not provide you with the level of health and energy that you're looking for.

Eating a balanced diet, getting regular sleep and sufficient exercise, reducing your daily toxic threshold, and maintaining a positive state of mind are required, as well. This may seem overwhelming at first, but I'm here to help you every step of the way. In weeks and months to come, after your first cleanse, you'll be able to refer to the book's index, the glossary of terms, the specific steps in the Oxygen Colon Cleanse program in Chapter 4, the diet suggestions in this chapter, and the Resources section, as well as notes you might jot down in any sections that seem particularly meaningful to your situation.

But first, you have to learn about your body and its processes before you can make healthy changes. So let's take a look at the biorhythms (or biological cycles) that regulate our bodies.

Leaning About the Human Body's Biorhythms

All creatures on this planet, including us human beings, are naturally attuned to three body cycles each and every day. These cycles have precise and established hours set by the universal laws of nature.

Body Cycle #1: Elimination

Your body's elimination cycle starts at about **4 a.m.** and ends at about **12 noon.** During this cycle the body naturally tries to purge itself of toxic waste materials and unnecessary salts, proteins, and acids. During this time it's ideal to feed the body adequate amounts of fresh seasonal fruit (preferably organic or locally grown). Not only does this supply the body with living matter to draw out and detoxify unwanted substances, it also ensures that the colon remains well hydrated and nourished. Fresh fruit provides the ideal environment to support the body's elimination cycle, since raw fruit provides water, oxygen, enzymes, live fiber, and vital nutrients.

Body Cycle #2: Energy

The energy cycle begins at about **12 noon** and ends at about **4 p.m.** This is when food and nutrients are processed and stored to provide you with the energy you need during the day. The best way to support your body during the energy cycle is to eat plenty of fresh raw vegetables (a salad, for instance) with a starch source, to help the body maintain its natural biochemical balance.

Body Cycle #3: Regeneration

The regeneration cycle lasts from about **8 p.m.** to **4 a.m.** This is an opportunity for the body to take the time it needs to heal and reenergize. This is when the body should get quality sleep. During this cycle the body assimilates and uses all the foods that it has stored during the day, and then processes their nutrients to regenerate itself, cell by cell. If the sleep cycle is disrupted by irregular work patterns, night feeding of infants, travel across many time zones, or other factors, the body loses its ability to regenerate the cells, which leads to *degeneration* of cells instead of regeneration.

What Is the Best Diet Plan for the Health of My Colon?

I designed the following general diet suggestions to fit the body's natural biorhythms. Understanding and following the principles below are critical for first improving and then maintaining your health and vitality. Although this diet may seem tough (at least on first glance), I would not be doing your colon or your body any good if I failed to tell you what they want and need to function properly.

For optimal health, all recommended foods should be *certified organic or locally grown.* This will help ensure that their purity and nutritional content haven't been compromised by toxins such as pesticides, antibiotics, hormones, and other chemicals.

Raw organic fruits, vegetables, seeds, nuts, and sprouted grains always provide the most nutrition to the body. Because they were not processed or treated, just gathered and cleaned, they provide the natural enzymes necessary for healthy digestion. Since we Americans generally were not raised on raw organic vegetables or foods, it may be difficult for you to make the transition from cooked, fried, and processed foods. Take it slowly and start by eating fresh fruit for breakfast every morning. After you've done that for a week or so, start eliminating one toxic food plus one toxic beverage every week until you have accomplished the goal of reducing your daily "toxic threshold." This process might last you several months, depending on how strict you are with yourself in keeping to the plan. In Chapter 6, I explain precisely how to eliminate toxins from the food you eat and the beverages you drink, thereby reducing your toxic threshold.

Drinking water or beverages with meals dilutes the digestive juices, which slows down the digestion process. Therefore, try to drink water only between meals, and don't use liquids to wash down your food in a frenzy of hurried eating. If this doesn't suit your lifestyle, limit your water intake during a meal to less than 8 ounces. I don't recommend drinking any other beverage except water during a meal.

You should *eat 5 times daily* to help regulate your metabolism. This might seem strict, but when you think about it, it really only takes a minute or two to peel and enjoy a banana, or eat a handful of seeds or nuts.

Eat slowly, and chew your food until it is a liquid before swallowing. This will allow your stomach to signal your brain that it is full, avoiding unnecessary calories. You produce up to 32 ounces of saliva per day—that's four 8-ounce glasses of it. Chewing your food will help the body absorb vital nutrients better and more rapidly due to the enzymes you secrete in your saliva. After food is liquefied in the mouth, the tongue will recognize the flavor of each certain food. The sensors on the tongue then send a message to the brain, which in turn sends a message to the digestive system resulting in the release of the correct digestive juices needed for that food. (Returning to the car metaphor we started in Chapter 1, this is a bit like an automobile assembly line that uses "just-in-time" practices to order and ship a part at the right time before it's needed.) Chewing your food well before swallowing ultimately leads to a more effective digestive process and is also one of the best-kept secrets for losing weight.

Does Any Combination of Organic Foods Create a Healthy Meal?

Consuming organic foods is a step in the right direction, though your body depends on the correct balance of food types. It's important to know how foods react with one another once they are inside the body. The real world of our eating habits has myriad food combinations, as well as many competing theories about the best combination to follow regularly. If any one person had all the answers, then there would be no need for me to write this book. So I will tell you what I have used, based on the biochemistry of the body and on what has worked for me in my practice and my personal life. Owing to space limitations, I will cover only the most damaging combinations of food, then I will present suggestions for five balanced meals that I'm sure you will enjoy.

STARCHY VEGETABLES AND GRAINS	NONSTARCHY VEGETABLES	
Bagels	Alfalfa sprouts	Mushrooms
Beans	Artichokes	Okra
Bread	Asparagus	Onions
Corn	Bamboo shoots	Peppers
Lentils	Broccoli	Radishes
Muffins	Brussels sprouts	Rutabaga
Pasta	Cabbage	Sauerkraut
Potatoes	Carrots	Snow peas
Tortillas	Cauliflower	Spinach
White rice	Celery	Summer squash
Winter squash	Eggplant	Tomatoes
(butternut, acorn)	Green beans	Turnips
Yams	Leafy lettuce	Water chestnuts
	Leeks	Zucchini

Mixing Proteins with Starches in a Meal Causes Colon Toxins

EXAMPLE OF STANDARD MEALS CONTAINING PROTEINS AND STARCHES:

Breakfast: Eggs, bacon, milk, sausage, or cheese *combined with* bread, potatoes, tortillas, and so on

Lunch/Dinner: Red meat, sandwich meat, chicken *combined with* baked potato, french fries, pasta, bread, and the like

When animal proteins and starches are metabolized, the end products are normally acidic. Your body should actually be slightly alkaline, not acidic. Your gastric juices contain three enzymes, which act on proteins, fats, and milk. They are pepsin, rennin, and lipase, respectively. Protein digestion requires an acid environment initiated by the secretion of pepsin into the stomach. Pepsin splits the protein molecule forming hydrochloric acid. As the stomach gains in acidity, while digesting protein, *starch digestion comes to an end*. We may say that those conditions, which are optimum for protein digestion, exclude starch digestion. Worse, the introduction of the starch almost neutralizes the acid, thus deactivating both enzymes and creating the climate for *putrefaction* and *fermentation*. *Nonstarchy vegetables* make for the best combinations with proteins. Refer to the food chart above.

Mixing Acid Foods and Starches in a Meal Causes Colon Toxins

Example: Bread, pasta, rice, and so forth, + any acid fruit or fruit juice

The digestion of starches begins in the mouth with an enzyme called ptyalin (pronounced *TIE-uh-lun*). Saliva, which is high in ptyalin, is secreted by the salivary glands and reduces starch to maltose, which in turn is reduced in the intestines to dextrose. Ptyalin will not activate in a mildly acidic or strong alkaline environment. The acid in regular vinegar, grapefruit, lemons, or other sour fruits will completely stop the action of ptyalin, resulting in a poorly digested meal. These meals will likely ferment, producing toxic by-products as well as decreasing the nutritional value.

Mixing Acids and Proteins in a Meal Causes Colon Toxins

Example: Meat + any acid fruit or fruit juice

Pepsin (an enzyme that digests protein) will act favorably in an acid environment. Therefore, you might think that the addition of *more* acids, such as citrus fruits, might improve the digestive process. This is not so! *The addition of citrus or other acids stops the secretion of the gastric juices necessary for protein digestion.* Either the pepsin will not be secreted in the presence of an acid, or the acidic environment will destroy the pepsin. Any acid eaten on a salad (say, vinegar or lemon), when eaten with a protein meal, stops the production of hydrochloric acid, since the pepsin interferes with protein digestion. An exception to this rule should be noted: Acids can be combined with nuts and seeds, because the high fat content of these foods will postpone gastric secretion until the acids have been assimilated into the body. Therefore, use raw nuts or seeds (not roasted or salted) with salads to neutralize the acids typically found in salad dressing.

Eating Meat with Cheese or Milk in a Meal Causes Colon Toxins

If two distinctly different high proteins (animal proteins) are eaten together, the amount of digestive secretions for each may serve to stop the action of the other. The body modifies the digestive process

HIGHLY ALKALINE FRUITS AND VEGETABLES (BEST OPTION)		OTHER ALKALINE FRUITS AND VEGETABLES	
Almonds	Grapes (sour)	Alfalfa	Garlic
Avocados	Kale	Apples	Grapefruit
Blackberries	Plums	Apricots	Honeydew
Carrots	Pomegranates	Artichokes	Horseradish
Celery	Prunes	Avocados	Kelp
Chives	Raisins	Bamboo shoots	Leeks
Cranberries	Raspberries	Beans	Lemon
Currants	Romaine	Beet leaves	Mangoes
Dates	Soybean sprouts	(snap, string,	Nectarines
Endive	Spinach	wax, navy)	Okra
Figs		Beets	Onions
		Berries (most)	Oranges
		Bok choy	Organic apple
		Broccoli	cider vinegar
		Cabbage	(organic)
		Cantaloupe	Papayas
		(red, white, savoy,	Parsnips
		Chinese)	Pears
		Celery	Pineapples
		Cherries	Pumpkins
		(both sweet	Romaine lettuce
		and sour)	Tangerines
		Chicory	Tomatoes
		Coconuts	Turnips
		Cucumbers	Watermelon
		Eggplant	

to the requirements of each food. Suppose milk was eaten with meat. This would initiate a highly acidic reaction, which would upset the proportion of pepsin and lipase acting on the meat. Both proteins would be incompletely digested, leading to the development of colon toxins.

What Are Some Alkaline Foods for Neutralizing Acid-Forming Foods?

Alkaline foods should be consumed 80 percent of the time. These foods aid in digestion, neutralize acids, and help restore the body's natural alkaline state. The foods listed above should always be eaten fresh, raw, or lightly steamed, and should be locally or organically grown. Although some fruits are classified as acid fruits, once they are broken down in the body, they convert the body fluids to an alkaline state.

General Recommended Diet Plan

Now that you've learned the basics about food mixing and optimal combinations, read on to find a ready-made diet plan that you can start today. This is no bland, uninspiring diet, either. The foods I've included (if prepared properly) are so loaded with energy and flavor, you won't ever want to return to eating the high-fat, processed foods we've become so accustomed to. Eating *five balanced meals* at the recommended times each day can help restore the health of your colon and consequently restore and enhance your overall well-being.

> **DOCTOR'S NOTE:** I recommend getting a full evaluation by your qualified natural health care provider, as well as having a food allergy test done. The Colon Diet is a general diet plan based on the body's biorhythms as well as my own clinical experience. Every person should have a custom plan, one developed to meet their specific dietary needs.

MEAL #1 OF THE DAY: BREAKFAST

Have breakfast between 4 a.m. and 9 a.m. Eat organic fresh fruit or drink freshly squeezed fruit juice. *Eat or drink only fruit.* Try to mix up the fruits during the week (but only one fruit per breakfast). *Example:* Do not eat bananas every morning. Try melons now and then, as they are one of the easiest foods to digest. Melons actually proceed directly to the intestines after being consumed. If they are held up in the stomach by other foods, they will decompose quickly and ferment. A melon is a great way to start the day. You can eat a different variety of fruits throughout the whole morning, but *never mix sweet fruits with acid fruits.* It's OK to mix sweet with subacid or acid with subacid (see below). Eat as much as you want until you are full. Remember, we are supporting the body's "elimination cycle."

> **ACID FRUITS:** These fruits have the greatest detoxification power: lemons, oranges, pineapples, strawberries, grapefruit, kumquats, tomatoes, tangerines, lime, sour grapes, and sour apples
>
> **SUBACID FRUITS:** Apricots, apples, pears, nectarines, sweet plums, cherries, mangoes, raspberries, kiwi, blackberries, blueberries, cranberries
>
> **SWEET FRUITS:** Bananas, papaya, dates, prunes, sweet grapes, cantaloupe, coconuts, mangoes, peaches, pears, watermelon, dates, digs, pomegranates, honeydew melon

MEAL #2 OF THE DAY: MIDMORNING SNACK
(Should be eaten halfway between breakfast and lunch)

For a nice brunch, you can snack on 1 of the following items: Choose A, B, C, or D. (For example, you might eat A on Mondays, B on Tuesdays, C on Wednesdays, and so on.) Remember to chew your food well before swallowing.

A—NUTS OR SEEDS: My favorite! It's said that a handful of seeds will provide the body with 12 to 14 hours of energy. Many people have reported that after eating seeds for their midmorning snack for three months, they noticed a 300 to 400 percent increase in their energy levels. Make sure your seeds or nuts are raw—roasted seeds have lost their life force For more flavor, you can mix in some hempseed oil, garlic juice, balsamic vinegar, or organic apple cider vinegar.

CHOOSE FROM AMONG THE FOLLOWING DELICIOUS SEEDS OR NUTS: Almonds, cashews, pumpkin seeds, Brazil nuts, pistachios, sunflower seeds, flax seeds, wheat berries, grape seeds, hazelnuts, pine nuts, squash seeds, sesame seeds, macadamia nuts, and walnuts. Siberian cedar nuts have one of the highest life-force energies and are the most nutritious and medicinally valuable pine nuts in the world; you can purchase these from *www.energyoflife.ca*. I also recommend that you read *Anastasia*, by Vladimir Megre, which will open your eyes and touch your soul.

B—ORGANIC SUPER GREEN FOOD SUPPLEMENT: Take a high-quality green powder mix, wheat grass or a chlorella supplement, in a 20-ounce glass of purified water and add 1 teaspoon of organic apple cider vinegar. This is fast and easy and provides your body with the nutritional value of five full salads.

C—ORGANIC GOJI BERRIES: If you're not familiar with the remarkable health benefits of Tibetan goji berries, do yourself a favor and give them a try. They pack more nutritional value into each bite than just about any other food.

D—ORGANIC AVOCADO: Cut your avocado and sprinkle with fresh-ground black or white pepper, then squeeze some fresh lime juice over it before eating. The pepper will speed up your metabolism. Avocado contains the enzyme lipase. Foods containing lipase (a digestive enzyme) are the ones that have naturally occurring "good fat." New research from UCLA indicates that organic avocados are the highest fruit source of lutein (a pigment that helps prevent eye disease) among

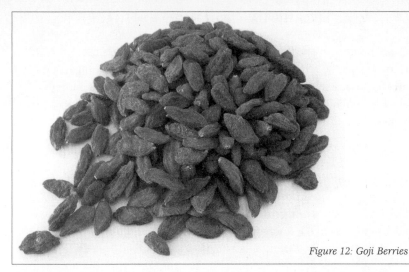

Figure 12: Goji Berries

the 20 most frequently eaten fruits. In addition, researchers found that avocados have nearly twice as much vitamin E as previously reported, making them the highest fruit source of this powerful antioxidant. Avocados also contain four times more beta-sitosterol than any other fruit, which helps lower blood cholesterol levels. Some studies have found that the avocado's beta-sitosterol content, combined with its monounsaturated fat content, helps it to lower cholesterol levels.

MEAL #3 OF THE DAY: LUNCH
Vegetable + starch

Have lunch between 11:30 a.m. and 1:30 p.m. Choose 2 to 3 alkaline vegetables (no acidic ones) and combine with a salad of fresh spinach, mixed lettuce, and greens (such as arugula, beet greens, or kale). Organic salad dressing or a mixture of oil and organic apple cider vinegar are excellent complements. Select only the red or dark-green leafy types of lettuce. Iceberg-type lettuces are usually hybrids and contain virtually zero nutritional value. Spinach (and baby spinach) is an excellent source of nutrients, and besides that it tastes great in salads. Mix some raw seeds or nuts of your choice into the salad.

PREPARE ONE STARCHY FOOD BELOW TO ACCOMPANY YOUR SALAD:
Potatoes (red, baked), cooked barley, beans, pumpkin, squash, Ezekiel bread, sprout bread, seven-grain bread, whole-grain pasta, lentils, millet, oatmeal, sweet potatoes, rice (brown or wild), rye, sauerkraut, chickpeas, beets, and cauliflower. If it can be eaten raw it is best, otherwise steam, boil, or bake.

MEAL #4 OF THE DAY: MIDAFTERNOON SNACK
(Should be eaten halfway between lunch and dinner)

These options will be the same as your midmorning snack. Choose **A, B, C, or D** (see the Meal #2 section above). (For example, you might eat A on Mondays, B on Tuesdays, C on Wednesdays, and so on.) Remember to chew your food well before swallowing, to get your digestive process off to a good start.

MEAL #5 OF THE DAY: DINNER
Vegetable + protein + fat

It's best to have dinner between 6 and 8 p.m. As with lunch, eat a large, fresh vegetable salad (with only alkaline vegetables) before anything else. Mix 2 tablespoons of flaxseed oil, or cold-pressed olive oil or hempseed oil, or grape seed oil, into your salad. This dressing will provide more flavor as well as the essential fatty acids that your body needs.

Although you need to pick one protein source for dinner, I strongly recommend that you avoid meat. If you absolutely *must* have meat on occasion, limit it to one serving per week, and *make sure it's organic.* Meat should come from animals raised without harmful antibiotics and hormones.

SOME GREAT SOURCES OF HEALTHY PROTEIN
(make sure they're *organic*):

Cold-water fish	Lamb
(cod, halibut, sole, haddock)	Legumes*
Cottage cheese	Rabbit
Other organic cheeses	Range-fed beef
Eggs	Veal
Fermented soy	Wild game

* Legumes include beans and peas, and can be a good source of protein if eaten with mixed vegetables (in a salad), or even if eaten with a complete protein (seeds, nuts, meat, and eggs). On their own, legumes are incomplete proteins and contain only certain amino acids.

If you want a little extra seasoning for your meal, Celtic or Himalayan sea salt are good substitutes for regular table salt. Braggs Liquid Aminos blend perks up just about any dish.

Make sure you don't overdo it at dinnertime. Let your appetite be your guide, and remember to chew your food thoroughly. You don't have to rush through your meal, barely tasting it and scarcely enjoying it. Choose good foods, prepare them simply, and then enjoy them. You are well on your way to better colon health.

PART II

The Long-Term Solution: Slowly Reduce Your Daily Exposure to Toxins

CHAPTER 6

How to Eliminate Colon Toxins from Food and Drink

As you pursue better health, it will be greatly to your advantage to take steps to eliminate common intestinal toxins from the foods you eat and the beverages you drink. This will take some thought and practice, but it can be done. Common toxins you can tackle include genetically modified foods, pesticides, meat and dairy, soy, white flour, table salt, MSG (monosodium glutamate), microwaved foods, refined sugar, artificial sweeteners, caffeine, coffee, and alcohol. At the end of many of the categories described below, I provide a quick reference chart, giving you easy-to-follow ways to reduce your daily exposure to these toxins or even eliminate them.

Remember, preventing toxins from ever entering your body is the real secret to health. Because we live in an addictive society, I recommend eliminating these toxin-producing substances at your own pace. Some people are gung-ho and eliminate everything at once. If you can do that, I congratulate you. In reality, though, it's easier to eliminate or greatly reduce two or three toxin-producing compounds every week. For example, you might start by eliminating microwaved food and white flour during Week 1, then tackle getting rid of soy and MSG in Week 2, and so on.

Every journey begins with a first step. You are now ready to embark on your transformation in health. So set some realistic goals, and be patient with yourself. Don't worry—I will tell you exactly what you need to do and how to do it.

Eliminating Colon Toxins from Food

Spend a few moments thinking about the foods you typically take in. How much of your diet consists of healthy, nutritious foods that help your mind *and* body to grow and thrive? And how much of it is made up of processed foods riddled with toxic chemical additives and preservatives?

Even supposed "healthy" foods such as fresh fruits and vegetables aren't always as safe and nutritious as you might think. With no thanks to irresponsible commercial farming techniques that depend on chemical fertilizers, pesticides, and hormones to grow bounteous crops on overworked land, an alarmingly large percentage of today's produce has become saturated with toxins and has lost most of its nutritional value.

In many ways, everything was fine until several decades ago, when big agribusinesses decided to start creating their own "improved" foods, mainly for profit reasons. When you take something from nature and manipulate or synthesize it, it loses its synergistic qualities and becomes almost useless—merely another foreign chemical or altered structure that our bodies aren't used to. It becomes literally *dead* or *toxic*.

The foods that nature grows overflow with life-giving energy. The foods manufactured to replace them lack this essential quality. It is impossible for these "fake foods" to give our bodies what they actually need.

The energy or life force in food is absolutely key to having a healthy body and colon.

If you can remember the formulas "*Live food = human life*" and "*Dead food = human death,*" then you have taken an important step toward achieving a healthy colon. How real is the difference between raw, living foods and dead foods that have been processed and cooked?

It's as real as the difference between a living, breathing cow munching grass contently in a field, and bloody cow parts wrapped in cellophane with an "expiration" date on a supermarket shelf.

Raw fruits, raw vegetables, seeds, nuts, and whole grains are all good examples of live foods. These are the kinds of foods that the human body depends on for energy to sustain and repair itself properly.

Dead foods are those that have been robbed of their nourishing vitality and laced with toxins, as a result of artificial conditions while being produced, processed, or prepared. For instance, the process of pasteurization uses heat to kill valuable live enzymes in dairy products. Without these enzymes (special proteins that living organisms produce), dairy products are virtually useless to your body and can cause allergies and chronic immune system overload.

If heat kills the enzymes in raw foods during pasteurization, then it makes sense that it would kill them in the foods we cook at home. It shouldn't be a big surprise that raw living foods, loaded with nutrients and active enzymes, are much, much healthier than foods that have been cooked to death and are devoid of any nutritional value. Fresh, raw foods such as fruits and vegetables help detoxify the colon and body naturally, and prevent unwanted disease.

More than half a century ago, in his book *Prescription for Energy*, Charles de Coti-Marsh explained: "By eating live foods you create a live body. Live foods contain essential nutrients the body needs to create and maintain energy. Dead foods advance age, decrease ability, and decrease energy...they are useless when dead, exposed to air, soaked with water or unduly dried."

Convenience foods that have been precooked, processed, or refined not only lack life-sustaining nutrients, they're also loaded with noxious (or harmful) chemicals that accumulate in the colon over time, leaving a hard, compacted toxic residue. If this toxic sludge sits in the colon long enough, these toxins will eventually work their way through the intestinal lining and back into the bloodstream, where they contribute to countless, lifespan-shortening diseases.

About now you may be thinking, "A good plan, therefore, would be to start eating lots of raw foods...right?" Well, yes and no. Yes, a diet of nutrient-rich raw foods is indeed a smart and healthy choice, but no, many of such foods today are losing their life-sustaining qualities.

Where Have All the Nutrients Gone?

Discouraging trends in mass agriculture are leading to nutrients being stripped from the land and, consequently, from the very crops grown on them. The problem lies with the condition of our ecosystems, our appetite for cheaply manufactured foods, our desire to consume many kinds of foods whatever the season where we live, and the advent of the genetic modification of foods.

Healthy ecosystems that support cultivation contain insects in the soil that crawl around, die, and constantly replenish nutrients. Nowadays, crops are sprayed with pesticides and insecticides that kill off the insects, thereby reducing the nutrients and poisoning our food.

Land should be given time to rest and replenish itself after certain harvests, allowing for nutrients to be replenished. Yet this is rarely practiced anymore. Huge companies are increasingly buying up farmland and using chemical fertilizers to crank out crop after crop, in an effort to keep pace with the consumer demand. The overall results of these profit-driven farming practices are toxin-laced crops having almost no natural nutritional value. Two decades ago a half-pound of spinach contained 50 milligrams of iron, but today it contains just 5. The typical potato has increased its niacin levels over the past 50 years, though it has lost 18 percent of its thiamine, 28 percent of its calcium, 50 percent of its riboflavin, 57 percent of its vitamin C and iron, *and* an astonishing 100 percent of its vitamin A.

DOCTOR'S NOTE: The Centre for Food Policy in London states that today you would have to eat eight oranges to ingest the same amount of vitamin A that your grandparents got from just one.

How Do Genetically Modified Foods Cause a Toxic Colon?

Poor nutrient content in soil is not our only worry. Now crops are being given new genetic material to achieve various results thought to be desirable. Experiments with the genetic makeup of diverse plant crops have led to resistance to pesticides, herbicides, and insecticides; enhanced levels of nutrients; and even tolerance to extreme weather conditions. Common products derived from genetically modified plants are cottonseed oil, soybeans, cocoa beans, canola, and corn. Genetically altered crops are taking over farmland at an alarming rate. Between 1996 and 2005, the amount of land cultivated with genetically modified organisms (GMOs) increased from 4.2 million acres to an astounding *222 million acres.*

In an article in *L.A. Weekly*, Margaret Wertheim expresses fears that "Quietly and stealthily, our fields are being turned into industrial factories. This is potentially the most dangerous technology since nuclear power, yet we have no way of finding out what is being done."

In 1994, the Flavr Savr tomato (engineered to resist rotting) was the first genetically modified food approved by the

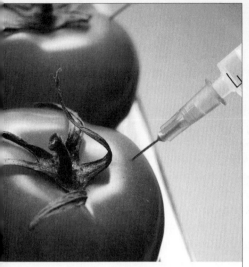

Figure 13: Tomato GMO

Food and Drug Administration (FDA) for sale for human consumption. Shockingly, FDA scientists actually warned that altered products such as the Flavr Savr could create toxins in food and trigger allergies, but they looked the other way and approved what some have called the "Frankenstein tomato."

HOW TO ELIMINATE TOXINS FROM GMO FOODS

1. Buy organic foods. Such foods cannot be grown using genetic modification.

2. Buy organic, range fed, hormone- and antibiotic-free meat and dairy products.

3. Avoid canola oil and cottonseed oil.

4. Corn and popcorn are usually genetically modified. Use organic sources only.

5. Use organic or locally grown zucchini and yellow squash.

6. Avoid all products containing aspartame, which is genetically modified and extremely toxic.

Why Buy Organic and Locally Grown?

But if we can't even count on our raw fruits and vegetables to be unadulterated sources of nutrition, how are we supposed to obtain the energy necessary for life?

The answer lies in choosing organically grown or locally grown (farmers market) foods. Even better, you should grow your own food organically in a backyard garden.

The U.S. Department of Agriculture (USDA) National Organic Program defines organic food production as "products produced under the authority of the Organic Foods Production Act. The principal guidelines for organic production are to use materials and practices that enhance the ecological balance of natural systems and that integrate the parts of the farming system into an ecological whole. Organic agriculture practices cannot ensure that products are completely free of residues; however, methods are used to minimize pollution from air, soil and water."

It's becoming more and more common to see organic fruits and vegetables at many grocery stores, supermarkets, and big-box stores. It's harder to find good organic meat, but it's well worth the search. Organic beverages are even available. Most likely, you can find a local co-op or farmers market in your town or just outside your town. This is the best place to buy your food because it is picked ripe, grown in your environment, and supportive of the local small farmers.

You might think organic foods are too expensive. But how much is your body worth?

How Do Pesticides in Food Cause a Toxic Colon?

Pesticides are used to rid an area of perceived "pests" such as insects, fungi, or weeds. Pesticides can take the form of chemicals, bacteria, or viruses. Used on crops to kill annoying invaders, pesticides can remain in the cultivated food products. When humans consume contaminated foods, these chemicals accumulate in the colon and slowly poison the body.

> ### FACTS ABOUT PESTICIDES
>
> ○ 94% percent of the residue from chlorinated hydrocarbon pesticides (such as dioxin and DDT) found in American diets can be attributed to meats, fish, dairy products, and eggs.
>
> ○ 55% of the chlorinated hydrocarbon pesticide residues found in the typical U.S. diet comes from meat alone.
>
> ○ 23% of the pesticide residue in the U.S. diet comes from dairy products.
>
> ○ The USDA tests fewer than 1 in 250,000 slaughtered animals for chemical toxin residue.

Despite international food standards set by 172 nations in 1963, seven of the most toxic chemical compounds known were not banned as pesticides in food production.

One commonly used POP (persistent organic pollutant), organochlorine, may be responsible for contaminating the world's seafood supply, since pesticides can run off the land into streams, lakes, and reservoirs. Organochlorines collect in fatty tissue and remain in an organism for a long time, and therefore fatty fish (such as mackerel, sardines, salmon, and albacore tuna)—normally a wonderful source of essential fatty acids (fats that our body needs and that we can get *only* from food)—are fast becoming unsafe to eat in regular quantities of two to three times weekly.

Because organochlorines break down slowly, they deposit toxic residue in the body over time. These harmful chemicals leak through the intestinal lining, accumulate in the body, and can cause headaches, seizures, skin irritation, tremors, respiratory problems, dizziness, and nausea. Many chronic conditions such as cancer, Parkinson's disease, neurological damage, and abnormal immune system function have been linked to exposure to organochlorines.

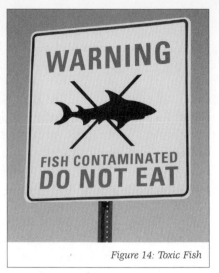

Figure 14: Toxic Fish

Will Washing and Peeling Help Reduce Pesticides?

It's always a good idea to thoroughly wash fresh produce before eating it, but doing so doesn't guarantee that you'll be able to completely eliminate all the toxic pesticides. The same goes for peeling. Also, peeling them greatly reduces their vital nutrient value.

HOW TO ELIMINATE TOXINS FROM PESTICIDES

1. Reduce the levels of pesticides you consume by 90% by avoiding these crop items: peaches, apples, nectarines, strawberries, cherries, pears, grapes, bell peppers, celery, carrots, and spinach. (If grown organically, they will be OK.)

2. If you are able to do so, grow your own food, using organic growing methods. This is the best way to ensure that you are not exposing yourself or your family to pesticides.

3. Cleanse your intestinal tract with oxygen two or three times weekly. This will prevent accumulated cancer-causing agents from leaking into your bloodstream.

How Do Meat and Dairy Cause a Toxic Colon?

Meat and milk, if left alone in their natural state, are not necessarily bad. But think for a moment about all the changes meat and dairy products go through, from the animals' birth, through their growth and the eventual slaughtering and processing for the table. When toxic hormones and antibiotics are injected into animals, they can be passed on to humans and can cause all kinds of health problems.

Hormones are naturally occurring chemical messengers that are produced by all plant and animal species to regulate growth. Synthetic

---

DOCTOR'S NOTE: People who eat just a hamburger's worth of red meat a day are 30 to 40 percent more likely to develop colon cancer than people who eat less than half that amount. Long-term consumption of three or more ounces of processed meats a day, such as hot dogs (or "mystery meat"), increased the risk of developing colon cancer by 50 percent.

---

hormone technology is applied to cattle farming to increase meat content and milk production. According to *Science News*, "Every year, about 30 million head of cattle are shipped off to feedlots where they are fed protein-rich fodder. 80 percent of these feedlot cattle receive steroid hormones, either in their food or through an implant in their ears, to augment muscle growth."

A large percentage of cows are also given antibiotics to counteract the rampant infection that spreads as a result of their confinement in overcrowded feedlots. Many calves are fed the blood of slaughtered cows, with little or no testing.

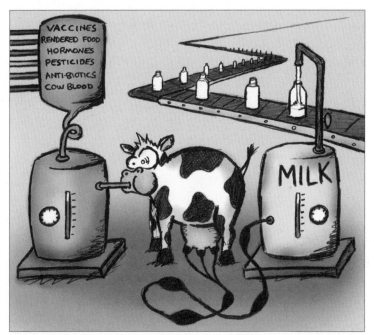

Figure 15: Hormone-fed Cow

HOW TO ELIMINATE TOXINS FROM MEAT AND DAIRY

○ Eat hormone and antibiotic-free, range-fed, organic meats or wild game. Buffalo and ostrich meat are good alternatives to beef. Limit meat intake to 1 to 3 meals weekly.

○ Eat more fish, but make sure it's free of pesticides and mercury. (See Chapter 7.)

○ Avoid processed meat at all costs—bacon, hot dogs, and sandwich meat.

○ Replace cow's milk with hemp milk, rice milk, almond milk, or raw goat's milk. Better yet, drink only *purified water*.

○ My personal favorite is hemp milk. It is delicious, with a nutty flavor, and provides essential and balanced nutrition.

○ Consume only organic cheese and goat cheese.

○ Whenever you eat meat, take an enzyme supplement, which will help your body digest it.

○ Chew each bite of food 25 times before swallowing, to mix it thoroughly with saliva and help take the burden off your stomach and intestines.

○ At each meal, eat more vegetables and smaller portions of meat.

Where do you think all these toxic hormones and antibiotics wind up? In the fat, muscle tissue (meat), and milk of the cows—and ultimately in the body tissue of consumers. *Cancer Epidemiology, Biomarkers, and Prevention* published a British survey that concluded the risk of colorectal cancer is increased by 12 to 17 percent for every four ounces of red meat a person consumes each day.

Another toxin lurking in the meat supply is nitrate, used to process and cure meats such as bacon, pepperoni, and hot dogs. When nitrates enter the body, they're converted to nitrites, which are extremely carcinogenic and can increase your risk of developing colon polyps. Studies have found that eating processed meat could make you two times more likely to develop colorectal polyps.

Beyond the sources of colon toxins in meat and dairy that include hormones, antibiotics, and nitrates, an even more shocking source is what is known as "rendered" food materials. Rendered food is what most people feed to their pets. It's also the medley that's fed to most of the animals that wind up in pieces in your local supermarket and then in your body.

How Does Soy Cause a Toxic Colon?

The reported health benefits of soy-based food products has led to a significant increase in the soybean's popularity in the United States. Soy marketers advertise its benefits regarding everything from heart disease to menopause. But is soy nature's miracle cure-all, or is its reputation just a bunch of hype?

One frequently heard argument is that soy plays a key role in the long, healthy lifespan enjoyed by the Japanese people. Why, then, is the life expectancy of the average American so much shorter than that of their counterparts in Japan?

Tons of products consumed in the United States contain soy. But the bean's popularity in the U.S. is a fairly recent development. The Japanese eat fermented soy, which is drastically different from the unfermented soy found in dry soybeans, soymilk, and tofu. By contrast, fermented soy products, such as fermented soymilk, tofu, miso, soy sauces, tempeh, and natto, may help prevent certain cancers and other diseases.

This benefit may be largely due to the fermentation process, which increases the amount of available isoflavones in the soy. Fermentation uses *live* organisms. Unfermented soy products in the United States not only are deficient in isoflavones, but also are full of natural toxins that can block enzymes needed for protein digestion. A large percentage of soy is genetically modified or is contaminated by pesticides, or both.

Mothers are advised never to feed their children soy-based formulas. In general, you are better off not drinking soymilk or eating soy-based products unless they were fermented. Read labels on dressings, which often contain soy. Products that contain lecithin or MSG, or that have "natural flavors," almost always contain soy. Avoiding processed foods altogether is a good way to keep hidden soy out of your diet.

How Does White Flour Cause a Toxic Colon?

White flour is a common ingredient made from the wheat grain. Unlike whole-grain flour, which uses wheat in its entirety (starch, protein, *and* fiber), white flour is made from only the starchy part. The healthy stuff is missing. In its place are usually synthetic B-vitamins that are engineered from petrochemicals derived from coal tar, which cause

---

HOW TO ELIMINATE TOXINS FROM WHITE FLOUR

○ Avoid foods made with white or "enriched" flour, which is bad for you.

○ Instead, use whole grains or sprouted-grain flour. These can easily be ordered online or purchased from supermarkets that carry natural foods. Grains should be soaked or sprouted for best results, to avoid irritating the intestinal lining.

○ Limit your white flour intake to two times weekly.

○ Do regular colon cleansing (two to three times per week) to relieve constipation and toxin buildup.

imbalances in the body. These synthetic vitamins are typically labeled as: thiamine (vitamin B-1), riboflavin (vitamin B-2), niacin (vitamin B-3), and calcium pantothenate (vitamin B-5).

Since white flour contains no fiber, it has difficulty moving through the large intestine. Processed foods, which often contain loads of white flour, can cause constipation and significantly increase waste transit time, thus giving toxins a greater opportunity to enter the bloodstream.

People who regularly eat white bread, white rice, and potatoes are at increased risk for developing diabetes. These foods can easily be replaced with whole-grain alternatives.

Carefully check labels whenever you shop for food. Many products that boast of having been "made with whole grains" were actually made from mostly white flour and contain just a small amount of whole grains. Foods commonly made from white flour include bread, pizza crusts, pasta, bagels, pretzels, crackers, tortillas, buns, and cereals.

How Does Table Salt Cause a Toxic Colon?

The Center for Science in the Public Interest (CSPI), a nutritional lobbying group, claims that sodium chloride, or common table salt, could be "the single deadliest ingredient in the food supply." There are two types of salt—good salt (living) and bad salt (dead and refined).

Salt is a natural antibiotic; it kills life, which is why it has been used as a preservative for thousands of years. By killing bacterial life in a food, salt slows the food's natural decomposition process. Salt also draws water from the bloodstream, causing the body to experience excessive thirst. These two factors, above all others, contribute to salt's damaging effects on the colon.

Refined salt's antibiotic properties kill off the beneficial bacteria that normally aid the colon in processing waste. At the same time,

HOW TO ELIMINATE TOXINS FROM TABLE SALT

○ Replace table salt with natural Himalayan salt or Celtic sea salt, which are natural and unprocessed.

○ Use Braggs Liquid Aminos to flavor dishes. This product is rich in essential and nonessential amino acids, and adds zest to meals.

○ For extra flavor, try using fresh herbs, lemon juice, or lime juice instead of table salt.

○ Cleanse your colon regularly to prevent constipation.

salt's dehydrating effects complicate the absorption of water, which leads to constipation and colon toxicity.

Most packaged and restaurant foods contain large amounts of table salt. Fortunately, the popularity of low-sodium diets has encouraged many companies and chefs to offer reduced-salt options. But be careful—there's a big difference between "less sodium," "low sodium," and truly low sodium. Natural salts are now being marketed as a replacement to table salt and are labeled as "sea salt," but be aware that these salts are also highly refined. On the other hand, products labeled "Himalayan Salt" or "Celtic Sea Salt" are living, were produced with ancient drying methods, and contain the vital minerals we need. Our body fluids closely resemble the makeup of seawater, so salts such as these are in fact beneficial for the proper balancing of our internal fluids.

HOW DOES MONOSODIUM GLUTAMATE (MSG) CAUSE A TOXIC COLON?

Glutamate is an amino acid that occurs naturally in foods containing protein, such as milk, mushrooms, and fish. MSG, or monosodium glutamate, is a manufactured flavor-enhancing food additive composed of only the sodium salt of glutamate. MSG is widely distributed in the food industry, and is most often disguised, with no product labels indicating its presence. Serious health conditions have been reported following the consumption of even trace amounts of MSG: asthma, headaches, skin irritations, gastrointestinal disturbances, allergies, obesity, diabetes, adrenal gland malfunction, seizures, high blood pressure, hypothyroidism, stroke, and heart complications. If you are experiencing any of these, it is imperative that you eliminate MSG from your diet.

HOW TO ELIMINATE TOXINS PRODUCED BY MSG

o Read all food labels at the supermarket. Avoid products containing MSG.

o When dining at a restaurant, ask whether the dishes contain MSG.

o Stay away from fast food restaurants. Most use MSG in their fries and drinks to make them taste better and to get you addicted to their foods.

o Cleanse your colon regularly to prevent the swelling of the mucus membranes in the gastrointestinal tract caused by consumption of MSG.

AM I COOKING FOOD THE WRONG WAY?

"I'd like the grilled chicken breast with sautéed vegetables, please." Most people would be proud of themselves for ordering that dish instead of the hamburger and fries. Unfortunately, it's not as healthy a decision as you might think. Because the vegetables are heated, their precious enzymes and vitamins can be lost or destroyed; they are no longer living sources of energy. Charles de Coti-Marsh maintains that a balanced uncooked meal "provides all the vitamins for the body's defense against diseases, anti-catarrhal factors, anti-ageing factors, anti-arthritic factors, anti-excess-calcium factors, sunshine vitamins, anti-sterility factors and rebuilding factors."

Let's consider the nutritional value of that seemingly healthy order of grilled chicken. Grilling meats, as well as barbecuing and broiling them, can actually produce HCAs (heterocyclic amines), which are known cancer-causing agents. As many as 17 different HCAs have been identified as a result of cooking meats at high temperatures. A connection has also been found between fried or baked starches and the formation of carcinogens.

HOW TO ELIMINATE TOXINS FROM MICROWAVED FOOD AND DRINKS

○ Ask all restaurants whether they use a microwave to reheat or cook foods. If so, request that your food be cooked by steaming, either on the stove or in the oven.

○ Replace your microwave with a convection oven.

○ Avoid cookware made of aluminum, copper, and stainless steel , and all Teflon-coated cookware. (Most stainless steel cookware contains nickel; 100 percent surgical stainless steel is OK.)

○ Cook the old-fashioned way—use simple, nontoxic cookware. I recommend glass, terracotta (without lead glaze), titanium, silicone, or cast-iron cookware.

○ Avoid heating beverages such as water and coffee in the microwave.

WHAT ABOUT COOKING FOOD IN MY MICROWAVE OVEN?

Say you want to heat up last night's macaroni and cheese, so you zap it in the microwave for two or three minutes. When you take it out, it might look like macaroni and cheese, smell like it, and even taste like it, but what you have is a radiated pile of zero-nutrient garbage. The microwave radiation inside the oven causes water, fat, and sugar molecules to rotate very quickly, thus creating friction, which generates heat. This radiation also destroys the chemical bonds that give these compounds their nutritional value.

But radiation causes ionization. A microwave oven decays and changes foods' molecular structure. Your body can't handle these irradiated molecules, and they eventually cause both your immune system and your digestive system to break down.

Right now, I want you to walk into your kitchen, unplug your microwave (if you have one), and get rid of it. Heating food in a microwave is referred to as "nuking," for a good reason. Nuked food is *dead* when it's pulled out of the microwave, and it's most certainly *dead* when it's put into the body. Remember: Your body wants to live. It needs foods that are high in energy, not high in toxins.

Now that you have looked at the evidence of toxicity at many levels of food production, processing, and preparation, are you ready to make some changes in your daily eating habits? You don't have to put all my suggestions into place today—getting your digestive system on the right track can't be done in a day or a week. Focusing on a couple of changes at a time, though, will increase your body's energy levels and begin building resistance to disease.

Eliminating Colon Toxins from Beverages

Unfortunately, many of the beverages we enjoy (or think we enjoy) create a highly toxic environment in our colons. Think about a can of soda—it doesn't have just one source of colon toxins, it has several.

A DRUG ADDICTION STORY: Instead of finding a drug dealer down a dark alley, a young boy buys his drug in the vending machine at his school, at least three times every day. He is innocent and does not even realize he has a tragic addiction to a powerful drug called a "soft drink." This drug is not only legal, it is freely available to him almost anytime he craves it. This boy has been addicted to this drug since early childhood and suffers daily from the side effects of depression, attention deficit, weight fluctuations, lack of self-confidence and self-esteem, fatigue, constipation, and anxiety.

The boy's actions are a cry for help, but no one hears it. When he comes home from school, he has access to even more of the drug in his family refrigerator: soda cans by the dozen, and more in the pantry. His parents and school teachers are teaching him not to do drugs, not to smoke, not to drink alcohol, yet they are feeding his addiction with one of the most toxic drugs of all time—refined sugar. By middle school, he is overweight, and newly diagnosed with diabetes, for which he is prescribed daily insulin shots as everyone stands around and watches his life slowly deteriorate. He continues this decline throughout the next few decades until, perhaps in his 40s or 50s, both his feet are amputated from the diabetes, then his legs are cut off below the knees, and then he suffers an emotionally and physically painful, slow death.

Moral of this story: You can change. If you start today to eliminate half the daily soda intake of you and your family, you are making great strides at beating sugar addiction.

The acids in your beloved can of soda may flavor or carbonate that soda, but also can irritate your colon. The sweet taste comes from either refined sugar (bad for you) or a sugar substitute (*really* bad for you). If your soda is caffeinated, it is even more toxic to your gastrointestinal tract.

Coffee, another caffeinated drink that Americans have come to depend on, really does a number on the bowels, as it disrupts healthy intestinal bacteria or flora. Alcoholic beverages are also popular sources of colon toxins. Sodas are addictive, and every kind is a drug.

How Does Refined Sugar Cause a Toxic Colon?

In 1998 the Center for Science in the Public Interest (CSPI) published a report aptly named *Liquid Candy*. It stated that "carbonated drinks are the single biggest source of refined sugars in the American diet...soda pop provides the average American with 7 teaspoons of sugars per day, out of a total of about 20 teaspoons." That's just an average. Today, a 12-ounce can of cola or soft drink actually contains 8 teaspoons of sugar. Commercial fruit juices can be just as bad; many of them contain only 10 percent or less real fruit juice, and the rest of the flavor comes from refined sugar and artificial flavorings.

Reading the labels of sweet foods and drinks can be confusing, because manufacturers will often mask sugar as something else. Don't let the following alter egos fool you—it's all refined sugar. Refined sugar may masquerade as processed fructose, corn syrup, sucrose, molasses, turbinado, sorbitol, dextrose, and others.

As long ago as 1957, Dr. William Coda Martin offered the following explanations: "Medically, a poison is anything applied to the body, ingested or developed inside the body, which can cause disease. Physically, a poison is any substance that inhibits the activity of chemicals or enzymes that activate reactions." Dr. Martin classified

DID YOU KNOW?

o The average American colon processes 100 pounds of refined sugar and 75 pounds of high-fructose corn syrup every year.

o Dentists are reporting that the front teeth of young boys and girls are almost completely devoid of enamel, caused by their drinking too much soda.

o According to the National Soft Drink Association, soda consumption is now over 600 12-ounce servings per person every year. Young males 12 to 16 years old are the biggest users, at an average 169 gallons per year.

o Soft drink companies gross over $60 billion each year selling this addictive drug.

refined sugar as a poison, because it has been depleted of its life force: vitamins and minerals.

When ingested daily, sugar produces a continuously high acid body pH. More minerals are then drawn from deep within the body in an attempt to restore balance. Finally, to protect the blood, calcium is leached from the bones and teeth in such great amounts that the bones start to decay and weaken, leading to osteoarthritis. Refined sugar consumption will damage the colon and eventually affect every organ in the body.

COLON TOXINS FROM ARTIFICIAL SWEETENERS

Artificial sweeteners are food additives that mimic the flavor of sugar but contain virtually no food energy. In the United States, the following five sugar substitutes are currently approved for consumer use: saccharin, neotame, acesulfame potassium, aspartame, and sucralose. Sucralose and aspartame are the most widespread and dangerous ones in use.

Sucralose can already be found in a wide variety of products. Surprisingly, many "nutritionally oriented" companies manufacture products containing sucralose, and many "health food" stores sell them. Has sucralose been proven, though? Does it provide any benefit to consumers? Does it truly "aid weight loss," as sometimes promised? Is it safe for the environment? Are there any long-term studies of its effects on humans? Unfortunately, the answer to all these questions is a resounding *no*.

Belonging to the "next generation" of high-intensity sugar substitutes, sucralose is sold as Splenda, a noncaloric, white, crystalline powder that tastes a lot like white table sugar but is 600 times sweeter.

HOW TO ELIMINATE TOXINS FROM REFINED SUGAR

o Replace refined sugars with organic agave nectar, xylitol, raw cane sugar, or locally grown unprocessed honey.

o Slowly eliminate soft drinks from your daily routine. Eliminate 12 ounces daily until you kick the habit.

o Avoid so-called "energy drinks" and store-bought "fruit-flavored juices" made from concentrate.

o Instead of sugary drinks, *drink purified water*.

o Limit sweets to three times weekly, and buy all-natural or organic sweets containing natural sugars.

o When you feel a craving for sweets or soda, eat some fresh fruit instead. This will help stabilize your blood sugar and satisfy the body's craving.

o Try mixing equal parts fresh fruit juice and club soda to create your own delicious soft drinks and punches.

o Drink unsweetened herbal tea with lemon, lime, or fresh mint.

o Cleanse your colon two to three times weekly with oxygen to reduce the acid environment in the bowel and excessive fermentation of sugars.

o Go through your pantry and refrigerator and throw out *everything* that has any of the following artificial sweeteners listed on the label: aspartame, acesulfame potassium (K), saccharin, or sucralose.

o Avoid the following brands: Equal, Nutrasweet, and Splenda.

o Avoid any product that claims to be "low-calorie," "diet" or "sugar-free," or claims to have "no added sugar." These all contain artificial sweeteners.

o Replace artificial sweeteners with natural sweeteners such as agave nectar, xylitol, or locally grown honey. Use organic sources if possible.

o Replace diet drinks with pure, clean purified water.

o Cleanse your intestinal tract regularly.

o Cleanse your liver and gallbladder to detoxify your body.

For more information on artificial sweeteners' toxic effects, visit *www. sweetpoison.com*.

Aspartame, most commonly sold as Equal or Nutrasweet, is another dangerous chemical food additive. At least 6,000 products around the world contain aspartame: "diet" carbonated and noncarbonated drinks, yogurt, pudding, tabletop sweeteners, gum, frozen confections, and even vitamins and cough drops. Aspartame has been linked to at least 92 documented side effects, such as muscle spasms, shooting pains, numbness in your legs, cramps, PMS, vertigo, dizziness, headaches, joint pain, blurred vision, memory loss, anxiety, depression, nausea, vomiting, diarrhea, heart palpitations, or seizures. Aspartame has also been linked to cancer, Alzheimer's disease, diabetes, hypertension, multiple sclerosis, ALS, and chronic fatigue syndrome.

How Does Caffeine Affect My Colon?

Caffeine is a highly addictive compound that many people have come to depend on for energy. It is found naturally in tea, coffee, and cocoa, and is added to many carbonated beverages, as well. Caffeine provides a "pick-me-up" by preventing the chemical adenosine from telling the brain to relax. The result is a surge of unnatural energy, but over time, the brain learns, and requires greater amounts of caffeine to provide the same increase in alertness—making it addictive.

Six of the seven most popular soft drinks contain caffeine. It's easy to get hooked if you're exposed to caffeinated beverages early on. With the addition of soft drink vending machines in schools, and

DID YOU KNOW? It's estimated that just one cup of coffee has more than 2,000 chemicals, many of which are gastrointestinal irritants and cancer-causing agents.

coffee shops on every corner, we are creating a nation of individuals dependent on this toxic substance. Drinking caffeinated beverages can dehydrate the body and interfere with the digestive process. Ultimately, caffeinated liquids will only slow the transit time of stool, causing fecal impaction in the colon. Caffeine also interferes with the absorption of magnesium, critical in maintaining regular bowel movements.

Coffee overstimulates the digestive system and can have a temporary laxative effect that can cause the bowels to expel waste before it's had the chance to process and use water and nutrients. This frequently leads to a constant state of dehydration and malnourishment among coffee drinkers. The same effects are seen in people who regularly drink decaf. Coffee is also highly acidic and can lead to an overproduction of stomach acid, which can severely irritate the intestines. Believe it or not, decaffeinated coffee has been shown to trigger even more acid production than regular coffee. To make matters worse, this overproduction of acid, when combined with coffee's laxative effects, can cause too much stomach acid to move into the intestines, potentially causing irreversible damage to the intestinal lining.

> **DOCTOR'S NOTE:** Slowly eliminating caffeine from your diet may actually relieve these conditions: irritable bowel syndrome, acid reflux, stomach ulcers, diarrhea, Crohn's disease, high blood pressure, ulcerative colitis, difficulty sleeping, and anxiety.

A lot of people think they *need* coffee just to make it through the day. But overcoming a coffee addiction is one of the best things you can do for better colon health. I recommend slowly eliminating coffee from your daily routine. Try substituting natural-grain coffee for your regular brew. Grain coffee is to coffee as herbal tea is to tea, and it has the added benefit of being naturally caffeine-free. Grain coffee is a ground mixture of things like grains, nuts, dried fruit, and natural flavors (this time *not* including MSG or soy). Such coffee is available for instant or regular drip coffee-makers. These substitutes come in a variety of flavors: vanilla nut, java, hazelnut, chocolate mint, almond amaretto, and the like. A great way to transition to grain coffee is to mix it with regular coffee as you scoop the dry grounds into your coffee filter. If you normally use 4 scoops of ground coffee, then try 3 scoops of coffee with 1 scoop of grain coffee for the first week, and continue to transition gradually until you have eliminated the regular coffee.

I don't recommend decaffeinated coffee or tea, since known carcinogens are used in the decaffeination process.

Do you have an addiction to caffeine? Try eliminating it from your routine for several days, then notice whether you experience withdrawal symptoms such as mood swings, headaches, and fatigue. Don't worry, though; the symptoms are only temporary and can be greatly reduced by drinking a lot of water and taking an oxygen-based intestinal cleanser.

How Does Alcohol Cause Colon Toxins?

Alcohol is another readily available beverage that poses grave health risks to human beings. It's estimated that over 100 million people in the United States regularly consume alcohol, and 1 in 10 drinkers has a notable problem with the substance. Alcoholic beverages disrupt a number of body processes, including those of the liver and the gastrointestinal tract.

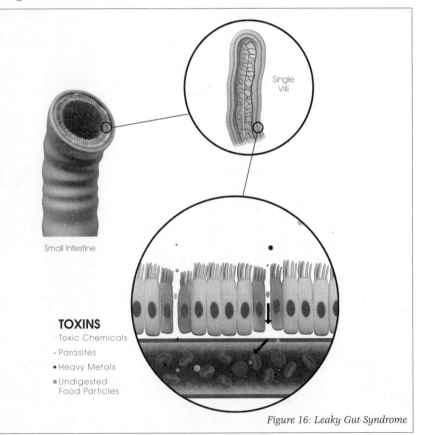

Single Villi

Small Intestine

TOXINS
- Toxic Chemicals
- Parasites
- Heavy Metals
- Undigested Food Particles

Figure 16: Leaky Gut Syndrome

DOCTOR'S TIP: Hangovers are actually caused by the dehydrating effects of alcohol, coupled with toxic effects of a chemical created naturally during the alcohol's fermentation or at some point during processing. Some drinkers claim that oxygen-based colon cleansers, if taken after drinking and before bedtime, reduce the effects of hangovers by up to 75%.

Alcohol is also a drug. If not treated, the effects can lead to cancer caused by permanent damage to vital organs; gastrointestinal illness, irritation, or ulcers; *Candida* or yeast overgrowth; sexual dysfunction; an overworked immune system; liver disease; malnutrition; and depression and anxiety.

Alcohol is also associated with gastrointestinal disorders, since it corrupts the mucosal lining and disrupts digestive enzyme function of the upper gastrointestinal tract, thus creating more hydrochloric acid than can be used. The stomach becomes inflamed, and ulcers form. Foods are not alkalized and acidic fluids wind up damaging the bowel lining. This can result in leaky gut syndrome, which allows undigested toxins to be absorbed into the body through the intestinal wall. Alcohol also impairs the body's ability to absorb many essential nutrients, including the vitamins A, B, D, E, and K, as well as calcium, zinc, and folic acid.

HOW TO ELIMINATE TOXINS FROM ALCOHOL

o Eliminate or drastically reduce all alcohol intake.

o Detoxify and cleanse your body. The cravings for alcohol will disappear.

o Reduce drinking habits to a maximum of one night per week. The safest alcoholic beverages are unfiltered beer or vodka.

o Drink extra water with raw organic apple cider vinegar instead of an alcoholic beverage.

o If alcohol abuse is a problem, seek help.

o Supplement with zinc and calcium (in the orotate form).

o Remember how alcohol makes you feel the next morning.

o Educate your children on the short- and long-term effects of alcohol consumption. Do them a favor and do not let them drink. Alcohol is a poison.

o Regular exercise increases your endorphins, giving you a "natural high."

o Take a good oxygen-based intestinal cleanser before bedtime on nights of alcohol consumption.

o Cleansing your colon weekly can reduce the effects that alcohol has on the intestinal mucosa, preventing leaky gut syndrome and the further fermentation of foods.

o To detoxify the liver of fatty deposits, I recommend three consecutive liver and gallbladder cleanses. (See Resources.)

CHAPTER 7

How to Eliminate Colon Toxins from Air & Water, Drugs & Stress, Metals & Parasites

As you read the previous chapter, you probably gave serious thought to reducing the variety of toxins you consume in all the things you eat and drink. You may already have started taking steps to combat them—if so, kudos to you! You may be feeling your health starting to improve, especially if you have done a colon cleanse (or two, or three) in addition to improving your eating habits across the board.

In this chapter, you will find out about other toxic substances that are literally all around you as you take a deep breath walking down the street, or drink a glass of tap water, or cook in a metal pan, or chat on your cell phone, or eat a dish of sushi at an iffy restaurant. As you learn about toxins that are everpresent in your environment, you can profit by following the tips I provide for reducing toxin exposure. (Also see the Resources section for additional products, services, and information.)

You are well on your way to better health.

Eliminating Toxins from Air

Try living without oxygen. It's the single most abundant element in our bodies, accounting for some 63 percent of our body weight. People can live for several weeks without food, and for about three days without water, but the brain dies after only six minutes without oxygen. Nearly half the world's oxygen comes from trees, grasses, and other plants, and the other half from ocean phytoplankton. Both sources are rapidly becoming exhausted by humankind's destructive habits.

The burning of coal and oil releases carbon dioxide into the atmosphere, thinning the protective ozone layer. An excess of ultraviolet B radiation is allowed through areas of the ozone layer that have gotten too thin. These rays infiltrate the ocean, interfering with phytoplankton's ability to produce oxygen. What's more, somewhere around the globe at least 100 acres of trees are cut down every minute, further depleting oxygen levels as well as allowing carbon dioxide levels to rise.

Exposure to an excess of carbon dioxide prevents red blood cells in the lungs from picking up oxygen and delivering it to other parts of the body. Oxygen is required to oxidize chemicals and other toxins within the body, which makes it an indispensable part of maintaining a healthy, functional colon. An environmental health researcher, Sara Shannon, theorizes, "We may have originally evolved in an atmosphere of 38 percent oxygen. Now, due to the loss of forests and ocean plankton, our two sources of oxygen production, measurements of oxygen as low as 12 percent and 15 percent have been made in heavily industrialized areas. This oxygen-depleted condition is a contributing cause of the generalized lack of well-being that many are experiencing."

How Can Air Cause a Toxic Colon?

The average person takes in about 30,000 breaths each day. Every one of them potentially does more harm than good. The air we breathe

IMPORTANT FACTS ABOUT INDOOR AIR QUALITY

○ Average Americans spend around 90% of their lives indoors.

○ Contaminated indoor air either causes or exacerbates over half of all illnesses.

○ Indoor air is up to 10 times more dangerous than outdoor air.

○ Most American buildings (homes, offices, and schools) are designed to be airtight, allowing pollutants to stay trapped inside and preventing the entrance of natural purifying agents such as ozone and negative ions.

○ Heavily insulated homes harbor more allergens than do homes with ordinary amounts of insulation.

○ Playing and crawling on a typical floor exposes babies to fumes from contaminants such as mold, mildew, and dust mites. One day of exposure introduces the equivalent of four cigarettes to an infant's lungs.

isn't just losing its vital oxygen content—it's gaining a number of harmful toxins. Remember that the colon depends on the body's getting enough oxygen to aid in toxin removal. How can the colon possibly eliminate chemicals and other poisonous material when the body is simultaneously faced with too many toxins and not enough oxygen?

By this point, you are already familiar with many of the common toxins we encounter every day in the outside world. The harmful effects of carbon dioxide, sulfur dioxide, and countless other chemicals bred by modern industries (mining, quarrying, transport, power generation, agriculture, and so on) are well documented. We know they're bad, but, realistically, an individual has little control over such aggressive and widespread pollutants. So, at least for the time being, instead of focusing on the obvious *outdoor* pollutants that drench our industrialized world, this section will highlight an array of less-obvious toxins that can permeate the air in familiar *indoor* environments.

The scariest part is the fact that *most of the toxins we absorb from the air come from indoor air*. Think about how much time most of us spend indoors—at home, at work and school, in stores, in indoor malls. These places are often havens for things like smoke, pet dander, paint fumes, mold, mildew, and dust mites.

The amount of colon toxins derived from indoor air is alarming. These toxins can be chemically based or derived from living organisms (such as animal dander or mold spores). You may be wondering how these airborne toxins get into your colon. Your airways are lined with mucus and, when you breathe, the majority of the toxins adhere to the mucous linings in the sinuses and air passages. This mucus, along with all those toxins, then drains into the throat where it is swallowed, transferring the toxins into the stomach and eventually the intestinal tract and colon. Some toxins are absorbed through the lungs and go directly into the bloodstream.

How Are Chemical Toxins an Indoor Hazard?

How can indoor air be far more hazardous to us than outdoor air, when refineries and vehicles emitting dangerous pollutants are all operating outdoors? Well, in outdoor environments, toxic chemicals dissipate through the air and wide-open spaces. But think about the nature of most indoor environments—buildings with four walls, a floor and a ceiling, and *maybe* a handful of windows that don't even open. Airborne chemicals literally get trapped inside homes and other structures with nowhere to go but into your body.

What Kinds of Chemical Toxins Can Permeate Indoor Air?

According to the EPA, "By volume, paint is the largest category of waste brought into household hazardous waste collection programs." Paint, especially older paints, can be extremely hazardous to the human body. If you have any old paint cans sitting around in the garage or basement, it's a good idea to get rid of them. Lead-based paints were commonly used until 1977, when the U.S. Consumer Product Safety Commission finally banned them, recognizing the risk of poisoning if consumed in the form of paint chips or dust. Mercury, also very toxic, was regularly added to preserve many latex paints until 1990, when the EPA banned its

HOW TO ELIMINATE TOXINS FROM VOCS

o Purchase nontoxic paints from alternative companies.

o Switch to nontoxic household products. Open windows or run exhaust fans every so often to reduce the circulation of fumes.

o Remove old or unneeded chemical products from your home. (Dispose of them at a designated drop-off place for toxic household wastes.)

o Read all product labels. Beware of products containing "methylene chloride" (such as paint stripper and aerosol spray-paint cans).

o Use a good air purification system that includes UV, negative ions, and HEPA filters.

o Avoid dry cleaning your clothes, or find a dry cleaner that uses natural dry cleaning agents.

o Always use a mask and gloves when handling VOC-containing products.

o Cleanse your intestines, liver, and gallbladder regularly.

See the Resources section.

use in indoor paints. A single breath of mercury fumes can poison the body and trigger a wide range of symptoms, including abdominal pain and diarrhea.

Now that lead and mercury have been banned, indoor paints are totally safe, right? Well, no. Most paints (even latex paints) release chemicals known as volatile organic compounds (VOCs) that can be extremely toxic once airborne. VOCs have high vapor pressures, which allow them to quickly evaporate and creep into the atmosphere. Millions of people are inhaling these toxic compounds each and every day, which can cause irritation of the eyes, nose, and throat; headaches; loss of coordination; nausea; and damage to the liver, kidneys, and central nervous system. Some VOCs have been shown to cause cancer in animals, while others are known or suspected to cause cancer in humans.

VOC levels are generally 10 times greater indoors than outdoors. Freshly applied indoor paint can actually produce up to a thousand times more VOCs. Yet paint isn't the only source of VOCs—in fact, tons of everyday products emit these harmful organic gases. The EPA provides us with examples of commonly used items: "...paint strippers and other solvents; wood preservatives; aerosol sprays; cleansers and disinfectants; moth repellents and air fresheners; stored fuels and automotive products; hobby supplies; dry-cleaned clothing, building materials and furnishings, office equipment such as copiers and printers, correction fluids and carbonless copy paper, graphics and craft materials including glues and adhesives, permanent markers, and photographic solutions."

Eliminating exposure to all products containing VOCs is probably impossible, but you can certainly take steps to limit your and your family's exposure to them in the household. The more toxins you eliminate from your environment, the healthier you and your colon become.

How Does Smoke Damage the Colon?

There's no debate on tobacco smoke's toxic effects on the lungs. It's common knowledge that the additives and chemicals in cigarette smoke cause lung cancer—but what's not so widely reported is the link between cigarettes and colorectal cancer. Tobacco smoke actually delivers carcinogens to the colon, as well as increasing the size of any polyps present there. This is serious business, since basically the larger a polyp becomes, the greater the risk of cancer. Smoking may account for about 12 percent of fatal cancers of the colon and rectum.

This one seems like an easy fix, right? Avoid colon toxins from tobacco smoke by...not smoking. Sounds reasonable, but unfortunately, the factor of *secondhand smoke* must be considered. Exposure to secondhand smoke, also known as environmental tobacco smoke (ETS), can cause toxic buildup in people who don't smoke, and may even lead to colon cancer by damaging genes. The risk of getting cancer from secondhand smoke is approximately 100 times greater than the risk from outdoor contaminants. This is especially unsettling in a society where one in four people smoke. The nonsmoker can potentially be exposed to tobacco smoke toxins in the workplace, at home, in restaurants, in public parks, and in other public places.

Fortunately, changing public smoking policies is not such a foreign idea. So far, 14 states have implemented significant antismoking laws—9 of these states ban smoking in nearly all places of work. This is encouraging, but we still have a long way to go. Children and nonsmoking adults continue to suffer from the ill effects of secondhand smoke in their own homes. Around 60 percent of children under the age of 5 live in a home with at least one smoker. Children are especially sensitive to secondhand smoke, because their developing organs are more easily damaged.

HOW TO ELIMINATE TOXINS FROM TOBACCO SMOKE

o Quit smoking. Hypnosis or a support group may help.

o Avoid smoking in the home.

o When you have the urge to smoke, distract yourself with an activity, a hobby, or a short-walk.

o Ask smokers to step out of the home if they must smoke.

o When going out to restaurants and other public places, make sure ahead of time that they are smoke-free, or at least have designated nonsmoking areas.

o Never smoke near a child, even outdoors.

o If quitting smoking is impossible for you, smoke all-natural or organic tobacco.

o Detoxify your body of built-up toxins with an intestinal, liver, gallbladder, and heavy metal cleanse.

o Repeat the following affirmation throughout the day: "I AM a nonsmoker."

Toxins from Biological Contaminants in the Air

The EPA defines biological contaminants as "living organisms or their derivatives." These include mold, mildew, bacteria, dust mites, animal dander, and viruses. Regular exposure to any of these can cause toxic buildup in the colon, which, as we know, can lead to the development of serious diseases in the body. Children, the elderly, and those with weakened immune systems are especially susceptible to airborne biological contaminants.

Many people commonly suffer from such outdoor allergens as pollen, cedar, and ragweed. At least as many people are allergic to a range of toxic biological contaminants found indoors, as well. Let's take a look at some of the most common indoor organisms, and then learn how to eliminate them from your environment.

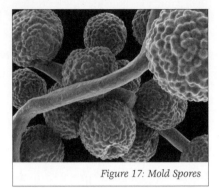

Figure 17: Mold Spores

MOLD AND MILDEW TOXINS IN YOUR HOME

Think about the last time you cleaned your bathroom, when you used a toxic bathroom cleaner to scrub nasty black mold and mildew off the shower tiles. Guess what? Your body was just bombarded with a slew of toxins—the chemicals from the cleaner itself, on top of the airborne mold spores you inhaled.

So what's the difference between mold and mildew? They're practically the same thing, and the terms are often used interchangeably. Molds are microscopic fungi that proliferate in damp areas, either indoors or out. Mold growing in a shower or bathtub is usually referred to as mildew. Mildew and mold reproduce by producing airborne spores that are constantly seeking more moisture. This is why

HOW TO ELIMINATE TOXINS FROM MOLD AND MILDEW

o *Controlling moisture is the key to regulating indoor mold.* Wipe away leaks, spills, or condensation as soon as you notice them.

o When necessary, use a dehumidifier to help clear moisture out of the air. If you live in a high-humidity area, dehumidify the house twice weekly.

o Run the air conditioner when needed, and make sure the filter is changed often.

o Ventilate the bathroom with a fan while showering.

o In Australia, tea tree oil is commonly used in ventilation systems to control bacteria and mold growth.

o Have your home tested for mold spores, particularly if you live in a humid area.

o Use a good air purification system that includes UV, negative ions, and HEPA filters. A germicidal UV lamp is most effective at destroying microorganisms like viruses, bacteria, and fungi (including mold).

See the Resources section.

DOCTOR'S NOTE: Molds may account for almost all chronic sinus infections, affecting 37 million Americans.

mold is found in sections of a home that are likely to have damp surfaces—walls (inside and out), cabinets, and any other poorly ventilated areas that can trap condensation and provide a breeding ground for mold.

Molds occur naturally outdoors, so it's expected that some airborne mold spores will make their way into indoor environments. The problem lies with the indoor mold colonies that multiply, releasing millions of spores that reach concentrations of hundreds of times higher than outdoors. Mold toxin exposure has been linked to respiratory ailments, as well as nausea and diarrhea.

COLON TOXINS FROM PET DANDER

Animal dander is similar to dandruff that humans can develop. Dander is just old skin cells that have come loose from an animal. Older pets tend to shed more dander than younger ones because their skin is drier, due to aging oil glands. Dander can accumulate all over the house, but is most concentrated in areas where the animal sleeps such as carpet, beds, sofas, and other upholstered furniture. When these skin cells become airborne, they're inhaled or swallowed, and ultimately end up inside *you*. Remember that virtually *all* the toxins you are exposed to every day enter through your intestinal lining.

Some 7 in 10 American households own cats or dogs, and 1 in 10 people are allergic to their animals. The Humane Society reports that about 2 million people with cat allergies actually live in a house

HOW TO ELIMINATE INDOOR TOXINS FROM PET DANDER

- If possible, keep your pets outside or in a designated room of your home. Place an air purifier in that room.

- Keep pets off the furniture and any carpeted areas as much as possible.

- Designate at least one room, such as the bedroom, to be "pet-free."

- Wash your hands thoroughly after petting your cats or dogs.

- Bathe your pet outdoors weekly with a high-quality, chemical-free pet shampoo. This alone can reduce pet dander by over 80%.

- Brush your pet outdoors three or more times weekly to reduce dander buildup.

- Change the A/C filter in your home monthly to prevent the recirculation of dander.

- Vacuum and wash all bedding frequently, using an all-natural laundry detergent, plus a vacuum with a HEPA filter.

- Use a good air purification system that includes UV, negative ion, and HEPA filtration.

- Cleanse your colon regularly.

DID YOU KNOW? Your mattress can host from 100,000 to *10 million* dust mites. They can account for 10% of the weight of pillows used over six years. Think about it: You spend roughly one-third of your life in bed.

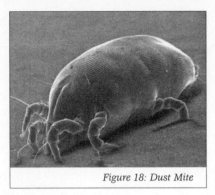

Figure 18: Dust Mite

with at least one cat. That's an awful lot of people who are needlessly breathing in toxic particles every day. If someone is severely allergic to pet dander, it is best to keep his or her environment as clean as possible.

COLON TOXINS FROM DUST MITES

Only a fraction of a millimeter long, the almost invisible dust mite permeates dust in houses all over the globe. Closely related to ticks and spiders, these eight-legged creatures live and breed in bedding, curtains, rugs, carpeting, stuffed animals, couches, and old clothes. Dust mites feed on animal dander, as well as the dead skin scales from humans. The life span of a dust mite is two to four months—in that time, it produces about 2,000 droppings.

HOW TO ELIMINATE TOXINS FROM DUST MITES

o Use a dehumidifier two to three times weekly in your home to reduce moisture. Dust mites are attracted to warm, humid areas, so try to keep the humidity under 50 percent.

o Use wood or plastic blinds and shades, instead of cloth drapes or curtains.

o Buy new pillows every year to prevent the accumulation of droppings, or use organic cotton dust mite mattress and pillow casings (available online).

o Wash all bedding weekly in very hot water (130°F.) with a natural laundry detergent. Add the essential oils tea tree and eucalyptus to the spin cycle when washing bedding, curtains, and rugs.

o Dry the washed items on a high heat cycle.

o Replace carpet with nontoxic hardwood flooring or nontoxic wool carpeting. (Or use all-natural dust-mite-killing carpet-cleaning supplies.)

o Vacuum often, but make sure people with severe dust allergies leave the house during the vacuuming. Use a vacuum that contains a HEPA filter, changing it often.

o Use a good air purification system that includes UV, negative ions, and HEPA filters.

o Cleanse your colon regularly.

These droppings are highly toxic, and when inhaled or swallowed they can accumulate in your intestinal tract.

Just one ounce of house dust can support some 30,000 dust mites. A study published in the *Journal of Allergy and Clinical Immunology* found that 84 percent of American homes contain detectable amounts of dust mites in bedding. Older homes, homes with mold, and homes with high humidity in the bedrooms usually have the highest levels of mites.

Research done at Clemson University reports that *dust mites are the second leading cause of allergic reactions*, the first being *pollen*. Dust mites are impossible to see without a microscope.

Let's Review

Daily airborne contaminants, such as mold, mildew, smoke, VOCs, dust mites, and pet dander, all contribute to well over 200,000 toxins entering your body every day.

Luckily, there are things you can do to improve the air quality of indoor environments. If you follow the suggestions I have given you, and slowly start protecting you and your family by eliminating these toxins, you can reduce your daily exposure to air toxins by a whopping 90 percent!

TIPS FOR CLEANSING THE AIR OF TOXINS

○ Place *live* toxin-absorbing plants in each room of your home and office. These plants can digest airborne toxins found indoors: Boston ferns, peace lilies, arrowhead vines, golden pothos, English ivy, spider plants, dracaenas, aceca palms, and chrysanthemums.

○ Use natural air fresheners, not chemically based ones. Dilute these essential oils in distilled water to spray around the home or office: tea tree, citronella, lavender, orange, and lemongrass.

○ Open windows slightly during a rainstorm to let fresh, clean, oxygen-rich air circulate.

Eliminating Toxins from Water

Water in our bodies helps keep things moving, decreasing the risk of constipation and maintaining regular waste elimination. Water is also necessary to help our body continuously flush toxins from the liver, kidneys, and colon. Equally critical is water's ability to aid in absorbing nutrients, particularly water-soluble vitamins. When the body's water supply is insufficient, the colon attempts to make up for it by sucking water from feces. Fecal matter without water—what does that spell? C-o-n-s-t-i-p-a-t-i-o-n. Stools will be harder to eliminate, and may irritate and even damage the intestinal lining. A chronically dehydrated colon will not produce healthy bowel movements, and can lead to other, more life-threatening bowel conditions.

Water is the secret to life. Every known form of living matter relies on water to survive. The human body is approximately 70 percent water, with the remaining 30 percent being solid matter. Both blood and the brain's gray matter are approximately 80 percent water. Our lungs, which are closely associated with air, are actually close to 90 percent water. Therefore, it's no surprise that we begin to feel ill, faint, or sluggish when our bodies are deprived of water.

Nearly all bodily processes require water, including digestion and waste elimination. Did you know that the amount of water we drink (or don't drink) each day plays a major role in whether or not we develop a toxic colon? Why is water so important?

Many people consume plenty of liquids throughout the day—but few people drink enough water. Drinking sodas and drinking water are *not* the same, especially concerning your digestive health. We're not made out of sodas, coffee, or alcohol—we're made out of (mostly) water. Drinking sodas or coffee throughout the day actually dehydrates the body and increases the amount of stress placed on the internal cleansing organs, such as the colon and liver. *Up to 90 percent of the population is chronically dehydrated.*

Sadly, even people who *do* drink enough water are often getting it from contaminated sources. The EPA lists over 80 "regulated" contaminants found in tap water, including chlorine, fluoride, arsenic, and numerous pesticides. The list doesn't include certain unregulated toxins such as perchlorate (a chemical found in rocket fuel).

You might be saying, "I don't need to read this chapter. I drink bottled water." But what about the toxic water that the cows, pigs, fish, or chicken drink that ends up in the meat you eat? What about the water used to grow the vegetables and fruit you enjoy? Or the water you yourself use to wash your dishes, clothes, and bedding? And what about the water you take a shower in or swim in? All these, and more, can expose you to toxic chemicals in water.

Drinking tap water overwhelms the intestines with toxins and prevents essential nutrients from being absorbed into the body. Even if you avoid drinking water from the tap, you're still exposed to toxins. Taking a shower for 15 minutes can expose your body to chemicals and the same amount of toxins as would drinking seven glasses of tap water. Further, the hot water of the shower makes your pores dilate and absorb all those toxins straight into the body. Similarly, if you're lounging next to the pool on a hot day and sweating in the sun, when you jump into the pool your skin, with its open pores, will absorb high levels of chlorine.

Unfortunately, we're not protecting ourselves by drinking bottled water, either. It has been documented that some of the major water "manufacturers" have actually been bottling tap water and selling it to the public. That means we can't always trust labels that read "drinking water" or "spring water"—they may not be as free of harmful chemicals as we thought.

Most Water Contains Arsenic

Arsenic is an extremely toxic, naturally occurring, heavy metal that damages the human nervous system, causes birth defects, and leads to several types of cancer. This substance is poisonous if inhaled, but the primary mode of contamination worldwide is through the water supply. The International Agency for Research on Cancer (IARC) has labeled arsenic as a Category 1 carcinogen—meaning that it's *definitely* a cancer-causing agent.

An article in *Toxicologic Pathology* in 2003 confirmed the link between arsenic-polluted water and the risk of developing multiple cancers, including colon cancer. The National Resources Defense Council (NRDC) estimates that over 34 million Americans consume water with a high enough concentration of arsenic to be considered carcinogenic. Arsenic enters the body through the intestinal tract where, if not eliminated, it can contribute to a weakened immune system and bowel disease.

Most Water Contains Fluoride

Fluoride is one of the most toxic substances known to science, yet the American Dental Association thinks that it's OK to put fluoride in our toothpaste. Even some vitamin supplements contain fluoride. In 2002 nearly 90 percent of the U.S. population was supplied by public water systems—of that, around 67 percent received fluoridated water.

Material safety data sheets (MSDS) label fluoride compounds as toxic chemicals that should be handled as such, by wearing a dust mask and goggles. *Fluorides are actually more toxic than lead, and only slightly less poisonous than arsenic.* Think about the toxins that your body must process simply from your brushing your teeth and rinsing your mouth. Fluoride compounds are purposefully added to both water (a process known as fluoridation) and toothpaste, to prevent tooth decay. Actually, fluoride has never been proven to significantly aid in protecting teeth from the development of cavities.

Every year, poison control centers receive thousands of calls from people reporting excessive consumption of fluoride-containing products (vitamins, toothpaste, mouthwash, and so on). Fluoride poisoning severely damages the body and can even lead to death. This lethal chemical in water creates a toxic state that can cause a range of ailments, including bone and uterine cancer, lowered IQ, birth defects and perinatal death, osteoarthritis, and gastrointestinal disorders.

Most Water Contains Chlorine

Another chemical contaminating water supplies nationwide is chlorine. Although a naturally occurring element, the chemical isolated from it is a disinfectant used to kill waterborne diseases such as cholera, dysentery, *E. coli*, and typhoid. It has regularly been used in municipal water treatment facilities for over a century, and more than *200 million Americans* (that is, two in three) have chlorinated water pumped into their homes every day.

While chlorine may be effective at eliminating many pathogens, its presence in drinking water may be doing more harm than good. When chlorine is added to water, it bonds with other natural compounds to form trihalomethanes (chlorination byproducts), or THMs. These chlorine byproducts trigger the production of free radicals in the body, causing cell damage, and are highly carcinogenic.

The *Journal of the National Cancer Institute* reported that rats developed tumors after being given water containing one of the same byproducts found in chlorinated drinking water systems. If animals are developing chlorine-related cancerous growths, then why are local governments continuing to pipe chlorinated water to citizens?

We also inhale chlorine in gas form and absorb it through our skin. Taking a hot shower contaminates the body with chlorine-treated water. Chlorine vapors from the bathroom can spread throughout the home, exposing others to its toxic effects. Inhaling chlorine is a serious health risk, since it's absorbed directly into the bloodstream.

Many nations recognize that chlorine is detrimental to the health of its citizens, and that alternatives exist for proper disinfection. The use of ozone O^3 in water treatment facilities has proven to be an effective practice for killing harmful viruses; some municipalities have switched to ozonation.

Most Water Contains Other Toxic Contaminants

Perchlorate is a toxic compound manufactured primarily to be an oxidizer in rocket fuel. It can also be found in fireworks, flares, airbags, and munitions. Do you want this in your body? Insufficient waste management procedures in the manufacturing of perchlorate have allowed the chemical to be released into water systems across the U.S. Contamination has been confirmed in at least 25 states. I believe this compound interferes with thyroid function and accumulates in the bowels, contributing to a toxic colon.

If you're getting concerned about the quality of the water from your tap, going out of your way to buy bottled water might seem like a worthwhile effort. However, studies conducted by the National Resources Defense Council tested over a thousand bottles of 103 brands of water, and observed that one in three was polluted by contaminants such as bacteria, arsenic, and synthetic organic chemicals.

Insufficient regulation can account for the shocking amount of bottled water that advertises purity but instead hosts a slew of contaminants. The NRDC reports that "the FDA's rules completely exempt waters that are packaged and sold within the same state, which account for between 60 and 70 percent of all bottled water sold in the United States." Bottled waters that have to comply with the FDA are not tested for contaminants as rigorously as municipal tap water.

By now you may be thinking, "Well, I might as well drink plain old tap water." According to the NRDC, that's often what you're getting in the bottle anyway. The council estimates that 25 percent of bottled water on the market is actually bottled tap water. Misleading labels fool the public into thinking it is being provided with pure and healthy water, when this could not be further from the truth. Most water bottles also contain phlalates and bisphenols (hormone disrupters and carcinogens), which may be leaching from the plastic container into the water.

DID YOU KNOW? The National Resources Defense Council observed a particular brand of bottle water with images of mountains and a lake on the label, which advertised its contents as "spring water." In fact, the source was a faucet in a parking lot next to a hazardous waste site.

HOW TO ELIMINATE TOXINS FROM WATER

o Drink water filtered by a commercial system, clean well water, or distilled water supplemented with raw, organic, apple cider vinegar.

o Test your water for contaminants (especially arsenic) with a home water test kit.

o Installing a whole-house water purification unit can eliminate over 99% of all water toxins in and around the home. If such a unit isn't feasible, install an undersink unit in all bathrooms and the kitchen.

o Install shower and bath filters—remember, your skin absorbs toxins.

o If you have a chlorinated pool, convert it to chlorine free.

o When buying bottled water, make sure it is packaged in glass.

o When traveling, take a good portable water purifier with you.

o Eat foods that naturally contain sulfur, including garlic, eggs, and onions. Sulfur helps remove arsenic from the body.

o Cleanse your colon regularly to prevent the buildup of arsenic, fluoride, chlorine, and other water toxins.

See the Resources section.

Is There a Solution?

You may be wondering what the point is of detoxifying your colon, and meanwhile drinking lots of water to maintain good digestive function, if the water you use is pumping toxins right back into your body.

We know that water is essential to digestive health, but our colons don't want cheap bottled water—much less water from the tap. We simply can't count on bottled water companies or our governments to provide us with clean water. There are far too many toxins present in our water to let us maintain an uncorrupted colon. It is up to all of us to do something about this.

For pure clean water, my recommendation is to drink *distilled water, Wellness Water* (from the Wellness Water purification systems), or *water from a well dug on clean, uncontaminated land.* Distilled water involves boiling, evaporating, then condensing the water, and finally storing it in a clean container. As the water is boiled, chemicals and other toxins are removed, thus superpurifying the water. The drawback of distillation is that it removes important minerals from the water, along with the contaminants.

If your goal is temporary detoxification, distilled water works beautifully to help clean out the colon. But if you regularly consume distilled water, it should be modified to meet the body's needs. Distilled water can recapture its essential minerals with the addition of a little *organic apple cider vinegar.* The process is simple enough for you to do in at home. I recommend the ratio of 1 gallon distilled water (preferably stored in glass) with 2 to 3 tablespoons unpasteurized, organic apple cider vinegar.

You can get distilled water at grocery stores and supermarkets. Apple cider vinegar can also be found at most stores, but it's often pasteurized. Since pasteurization involves heating the product, the process kills the life force of the vinegar, so buy only *unpasteurized* (raw) organic apple cider vinegar. You can find it at grocery stores with a natural foods section, or at health food stores, and online.

Raw apple cider vinegar has been used for centuries as a remedy for all kinds of health issues, including colon cleansing. It contains vital enzymes that the body needs, as well as bacteria that naturally aid in colon function. Raw apple cider vinegar helps regulate your pH (the acidity and alkalinity of your body) and reduces the chance of constipation, which in turn lessens your risk of developing a toxic colon.

Eliminating Toxins from Prescription Drugs

Consider the following scenario: Ms. Rivera has been experiencing a chronic headache for weeks. So she goes to her doctor, a trusted professional, in hopes of finding a way to get rid of it. "Doctor, I've had a headache for some time now. It's wearing me down." "No, problem, Ms. Rivera. We'll get you fixed up," she replies. Five minutes later, Ms. Rivera walks out of the exam room with a slip of paper in hand. She drops by the pharmacy, and arrives home with her prescription pain medication.

The pills cover up the pain, but a month later Ms. Rivera has to visit her doctor again. "Doctor, I haven't been having any bowel movements lately, and my stomach really hurts." The doctor says, "Oh, did I forget to mention that the pain medication can cause constipation and possible stomach ulcers? Don't worry, though. We'll get you fixed up." Five minutes later, Ms. Rivera walks out of the exam room with a new prescription. When she gets home, she takes her pill for headache pain, a pill for constipation, and now a pill for her stomach ulcer.

What's wrong with this picture? First, the doctor spent only about five minutes with her patient. The average time a physician spends with a patient is now seven minutes—not nearly enough time to diagnose a patient correctly and come up with a treatment plan. Second, the doctor automatically prescribed a drug without asking any further questions of her patient or considering alternatives. Ms. Rivera walked in with a headache, and the doctor's only choices were to prescribe a drug for it, do surgery on it, or radiate it—that is, drug it, cut it, or burn it. The pain medication *did* cover the pain, but it was merely a bandage—it didn't address the root cause.

In our scenario, perhaps the source of the patient's pain was too much coffee and a lot of stress, or a bone out of position in the neck, or an eyesight problem that caused the headache. Who knows? The doctor didn't take the time to find out. She prescribed a pill that masked the headache but damaged the digestive tract. As a result, Ms. Rivera ended up taking three medications for a simple headache. Think about the combined amount of toxic residue from these synthetic pharmaceuticals that's now burdening her body—all unnecessary.

Aren't Prescription Drugs Supposed to Fix What's Wrong?

Nearly half of all American citizens take at least one prescription medication, and about one in five people take three or more medications. Pharmaceutical drugs are synthetic. They pollute the body, contribute to colon toxicity, and suppress the immune system. It's sad that pharmaceuticals have become the quick and easy solution to health problems, when, ironically, most of these "medicines" actually interfere with healthy bodily function. Consequences of relying on pharmaceuticals are weight gain, constipation, cancer, kidney disease, heart failure, depression, and more.

The colon is one of many organs negatively influenced by the consumption of prescription drugs. Constipation is a common result of taking certain medications. While many people might think it a small price to pay for alleviating their condition, remember that constipation is extremely unhealthy, especially if prolonged, and may eventually cause colorectal cancer.

ALARMING STATISTICS

o Illegible prescriptions account for over 7,000 American deaths every year.

o Every year, more than 2 million people suffer adverse reactions to prescription drugs while in the hospital.

o Every year, around 20 million people are mistakenly prescribed antibiotics for viral infections.

o Unnecessary medical procedures and prescriptions account for 783,936 American deaths annually. In 2001, heart disease accounted for only 699,697 deaths, and cancer for 553,251.

o Over 700,000 Americans wind up in the emergency room every year due to prescription drug overdoses and other adverse drugs events.

DRUGS THAT CAN CAUSE CONSTIPATION

Antacids containing aluminum	Calcium channel blockers
Anticonvulsants	Decongestants
Antidepressants	Diuretics
Antidiarrheal agents	Iron supplements
Antihistamines	Muscle relaxers
Anti-inflammatories	Narcotics
Antipsychotics	Parkinson's disease drugs
Antispasmodics	Sedatives
Beta blockers	Tranquilizers

CAN ANTIBIOTICS DAMAGE MY COLON?

Antibiotics are drugs that destroy bacteria or inhibit their growth, and are possibly the most overprescribed medications. If overused, they can kill the "good" gut bacteria, cause diarrhea and colitis, and lead to antibiotic resistance. Commonly, viral infections are misdiagnosed as bacterial infections—in these cases, patients receive a completely pointless dose of antibiotics. Over 3 million pounds of antibiotics are prescribed every year. Whether the prescriptions are necessary or not, those antibiotic drugs are contaminating intestinal tracts and causing serious side effects.

"Good" bacteria—also referred to as friendly bacteria, healthy bacteria, gut flora, or intestinal flora—take residence in a baby's colon shortly after birth. Trillions of these bacteria live, multiply, and help fight infection throughout its life. Although a small number of unhealthy bacteria are present in a baby, they are far outnumbered by the good bacteria that keep them in check. However, antibiotics can reduce the number of healthy bacteria in the gut, making room for the bad bacteria and *Candida* to thrive.

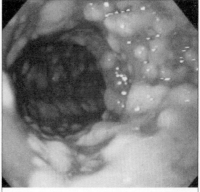

Figure 19: Clostridium

Clostridium difficile is the most common "bad bacteria" that multiplies in the colon if antibiotics kill off the friendly bacteria. It produces a toxin

DOCTOR'S NOTE: If you *must* take antibiotics, use a natural probiotic formula as well, to replenish the good gut bacteria. I recommend the Bacillus Laterosporus strain, or Bacillus Sporogenes, to quickly restore bowel health.

that builds up in the colon, causes diarrhea, and sometimes severely damages the colon's lining. This condition is known variously as antibiotic-associated diarrhea, antibiotic-associated colitis, pseudomembranous colitis, or *Clostridium difficile* colitis.

ARE VACCINATIONS BAD FOR THE COLON?

Vaccines have long been controversial. Although there are serious diseases out there, the risk of vaccination side effects really does outweigh the benefits. These drugs overload the immune system with toxins and depress its function, making the body more susceptible to developing a range of other diseases.

Did your doctor explain the risks to you before he stuck you or your child? Many vaccines contain harmful (even lethal) ingredients that damage the colon and other organs in the body. These include formaldehyde, spermicide, cancer-causing agents, gelatin from butchered animals, foreign DNA/RNA fragments, live viruses, mercury, and various antibiotics.

You have options to taking vaccines and pharmaceutical drugs. Talk to your natural health care practitioner about alternatives.

Eliminating Toxins from Stress

Whether it's physical, emotional, or spiritual, stress is responsible for creating or exacerbating many intestinal ailments, as

HOW TO ELIMINATE TOXINS FROM PRESCRIPTION DRUGS

o Start with doing an Oxygen Colon Cleanse (see Chapter 4), followed by doing three back-to-back liver and gallbladder cleanses, plus a parasite and heavy metal cleanse. Drug residue collects in the liver, which should be flushed at least every six months, even if you take no drugs at all. *Caution:* Time-contingent detoxification is a slow process of weaning you off drugs slowly, so talk with your doctor before discontinuing any medications.

o If drug abuse is an issue, structured intervention may be the best solution. Find a rehab center that specializes in cleansing *and* counseling.

o Ask your natural health care practitioner about natural alternatives.

o Cleanse your colon regularly to flush toxic drugs out of your system and prevent intestinal damage.

o Take probiotics regularly to replenish the bowels' good bacteria.

See Resources.

well as making the body less capable of protecting itself from disease. The widespread effects of stress are progressively weakening the health of many.

Common symptoms include headaches, heart palpitations, insomnia, sexual dysfunction, fatigue, poor memory, irritability, muscle aches, compulsive eating, grinding teeth, impatience, anger, depression, indigestion, constipation, bossiness, constant worry, anxiety, crying often, or excessive alcohol consumption.

Stress is a highly personal thing. What's stressful for one person may be neutral or even relaxing for another. It's important that you know yourself well and understand the limits of your body and mind. Although stress has come to have a negative connotation in recent years, we sometimes forget that *there is good stress*, as well. Good stress (or "eustress"), which results in feelings of excitement or fulfillment, can help an individual complete tasks effectively and efficiently.

Researchers have found that brief spurts of stress can actually help to fortify the immune system. It's the prolonged, bad stress (or "distress") that you have to worry about. Bad stress can manifest itself in fear, anger, anxiety, depression, or many other forms. Chronic levels of any of these negative emotions can cause stress hormones to accelerate or inhibit the movement of wastes through the colon. Over time, this can increase appetite and lead to unwanted weight gain. The colon is extremely sensitive to stress responses.

FACTS ABOUT THE STRESS EPIDEMIC

- Three in four Americans experience stress once a week.

- Half of all stressed people suffer from elevated stress levels at least every other week.

- One in six Americans experiences harmful stress at work.

- One in four prescriptions written are for tranquilizers, antidepressants, and anti-anxiety medications.

- Stress is linked to alcoholism, obesity, drug addiction, and suicide.

- Over half of all deaths occurring before the age of 65 can be attributed to stressful lifestyles.

How Is Stress Related to a Toxic Colon?

When people are busy and stressed, they tend not to take care of their bodies. In the hustle and bustle of life and work and family duties, many people put off going to the bathroom. Delaying a bowel movement is one of the most common reasons that people become constipated, which in turn leads to a toxic colon. A stressful schedule can also lead many people to eat on the run. Most fast-food diets include large portions of meat, fat, and sugar and very few portions of vegetables, whole grains, and water. This type of low-fiber food, if eaten regularly, can lead to both stress and a backed-up, toxic colon.

Stressed individuals also skip meals or eat hurriedly, not taking the time to chew their food. While a regular eating schedule leads to regular bowel movements, inconsistent or rushed meals can lead to constipation as well as other problems in the gut.

Constipation itself can be a direct result of stress-related changes in the nervous system. Normal bowel movements are produced after a set of complicated signals sent by the nervous system. Too much stress can cause an interruption of these signals and inhibit intestinal motility, resulting in irregular bowel movements.

Since bad stress is toxic to the overall health of the colon, what happens if you add lack of exercise and lack of sleep to the picture? Now it's not looking good. Humans are designed to be on the move, not on the couch. A typical American watches about six hours of television every day, and works at a sedentary job. Rarely do they make time to exercise when they get home. It's no surprise that the U.S. has become one of the fattest nations in the world.

Exercise gives power to the lymphatic system. Major roles of that system are to manage waste, help deliver nutrients, and remove toxic waste from cells. If it isn't functioning properly, toxins can accumulate and further poison the body. If the body remains in a toxic state, depression can ensue. Depression is one of those negative emotions that puts unneeded stress on the colon, and can make a person less likely to exercise. The benefits of exercise are not just limited to the lymphatic system. A study published by Texas Tech University reports that "regular exercise reduces the risk of developing colon cancer and the risk of death from colon cancer." The muscles in the colon benefit from regular exercise, and contribute to healthy bowel movements. Lack of exercise causes these muscles to weaken, making it difficult to eliminate wastes efficiently. Exercise also boosts the immune system, which helps protect against developing diseases of the colon.

Inadequate sleep can compound the effects of stress and contribute to a toxic colon. Not catching enough Z's at night may disrupt appetite-regulating hormones and cause individuals to overeat. Overeating, in turn, can lead to obesity, a major risk factor for colon cancer. It's also speculated that people make less-healthy dietary choices when sleep-deprived. Filling the body with unhealthy food leads to toxins accumulating in the colon and a lack of nutrients for it to absorb. Studies indicate that a shortage of sleep also causes the body to produce more stress hormones, which aggravate irritable bowel syndrome and can cause constipation.

Can Stress from Trauma Cause Colon Malfunction?

Physical stress can also take a toll on the body. Trauma (such as pain after a car accident or surgery), chronic work-related stress (such as lifting heavy objects or working long hours), too *much* exercise, and spinal misalignment can all overstress the colon and impair digestive processes. Americans are notorious for working long hours, when workers in many other (often healthier) industrialized countries put in fewer hours on the job; Americans get far less vacation time. It's no wonder we're having so many stress-related problems—there's no time to allow the body to regenerate. Physical stress due to overexertion also may lead to psychological or emotional stress.

A less obvious physical stressor is a misaligned spine. Injury or abnormal growth patterns in the spine sometimes result in vertebrae misalignment, referred to as a subluxation, which stresses spinal discs, joints, and muscles. The nervous system may also become aggravated, which can hinder organ functions all over the body. The first lumbar nerve (in the lower back) controls the opening and closing of the ileocecal valve and regulates the colon's contractions. A misalignment of the L1 vertebra affects the intestinal tract, resulting in constipation, diarrhea, and colitis. Hemorrhoids have been linked to a misalignment of the coccyx (tailbone). Intestinal malfunction can affect the gallbladder, liver, stomach, pancreas, appendix, and rectum. A chiropractic spinal realignment can benefit anyone affected by stress, since the nervous system is controlled by spinal impulses. I recommend that everyone get at least one spinal alignment every month.

Life is demanding, and some level of stress is to be expected. On average, toxins from stress affect your colon daily. This is enough cause for concern, but chronic levels are even more debilitating and can introduce greater amounts of toxins into your body. The colon is highly sensitive to your stress levels, so you should take measures to minimize the amount of stress that you experience day to day.

HOW TO ELIMINATE TOXINS FROM STRESS

THE POWER OF MEDITATION: Calming the mind is one of the fastest ways to eliminate stress and negative emotions. Sit quietly, eyes closed, and don't think at all. Sit comfortably, preferably early in the morning and outside. Feel yourself, the trees, the sky, the infinite universe as one. To learn meditation methods, go online or visit a bookstore.

THE POWER OF CHIROPRACTIC: Get regular adjustments from a chiropractor to keep the nerve pathways to the bowels functioning properly and relieve stress.

THE POWER OF MUSIC: Music can help relieve stress. Go online for many stress-relieving CDs.

THE POWER OF EXERCISE: Exercise increases stress-relieving endorphins and also promotes healthy digestion. It may seem yet one more thing to add to your schedule, but it will be worth it. I recommend rebounding (mini-trampoline) for stress relief and toxin removal.

THE POWER OF LAUGHTER: Sounds corny but it works. Look at yourself in a mirror and start laughing at yourself. Keep going and soon you will forget what you are stressed about.

THE POWER OF MASSAGE: Massage is a great way to relieve tension and relax the body. Try to get a massage at least once a week. If you can't afford a massage, touching and hugging both relax the body. Hug someone for a couple of minutes, and see how you feel.

THE POWER OF CHANGE: Examine what is causing you stress, and change those factors in your life. If you don't enjoy your life the way it is, then make adjustments so you can become the person you want to be. Resisting change will only make you stagnant.

THE POWER OF SLEEP: Most people don't get enough deep, restful sleep. If you need help sleeping, try natural sleep patches.

THE POWER OF NATURE AND THE SUN: If you live where it's convenient to take walks in nature, this is best. Getting even 20 minutes in the sun in the morning will energize you. In the evening, it can help you wind down and relax. Placing a small waterfall in your office or home will help relieve tension and remind you of nature's calming effects and beauty.

THE POWER OF LOVE: Create a "Space of Love" for you and your family, as well as an organic garden to relieve stress. Read the *Anastasia* series of books by Vladimir Megre.

THE POWER OF COLOR: Dark blue has a calming effect on the body. Try wearing a dark-blue shirt or blouse on days you know will be stressful.

AROMATHERAPY: The benefits of aromatherapy date back thousands of years. Stress-relieving essential oils include lavender, jasmine, chamomile, geranium, and lemongrass. Place several drops in the palm of your hand, rub hands together, and cup hands over nose, inhaling deeply 9 times.

EFT AND NLP: Emotional Freedom Techniques and Neurolinguistic Programming are both techniques that can help you relieve stress. Find a practitioner in your area.

Eliminating Intestinal Toxins from Heavy Metals

When you last drank a canned beverage, put on deodorant, ate some fish, or had a cavity filled, you exposed your body to toxins from metals. The canned drink and the deodorant contain aluminum, and mercury is a component of dental fillings—both are extremely toxic. Humans and other organisms do need small amounts of the *heavy metals* zinc, cobalt, manganese, molybdenum, vanadium, copper, and strontium, but in excess these elements can damage the body.

DID YOU KNOW? Your body may be exposed daily to toxic metals from: cosmetics, pharmaceuticals, hygiene products, food and beverage storage containers, paints, cigarettes, and many more.

The real health concern is the more than 20 heavy metals in use today that our biological systems simply don't need. We're exposed to their toxins via ingestion, inhalation, and skin or eye contact. Once in the body, heavy metals multiply harmful free radicals (by up to a million times) and cause damaging chain reactions. This poisons the body; impairs the function of cells, tissues, and organs; and can lead to cancer as well as countless other forms of disease.

BE AWARE: Many herbal supplements contain levels of heavy metals that exceed federal drinking water standards by 10 to 20 times. These supplements are cheaply made and sold at drugstores, supermarkets, and discount stores. Spend the extra money and buy quality supplements.

Four common metals in particular can damage the intestinal tract and contribute to colon toxicity. On the Top 20 Hazardous Substances list of the Agency for Toxic Substances and Disease Registry, lead appears second, mercury third, and cadmium eighth.

LEAD is the second most hazardous substance and is found in a number of products, including fuel, ammunition, pencils, pesticides, X-ray shields, weights, and cigarettes. Exposure to it most often occurs when airborne particulates and paints containing lead contaminate drinking water through corroded pipes. Tobacco smoke can contain dangerous amounts of lead. Lead poisoning can result in symptoms such as abdominal pain and constipation.

MERCURY (both organic and inorganic) is highly toxic, and both can seriously harm the colon. Inorganic mercury is used in thermometers, thermostats, dental amalgam (fillings), batteries, barometers, skin-tightening creams, various pharmaceutical drugs (laxatives, diuretics, and antiseptics), vaccines, and pesticides. Inhalation of inorganic mercury vapors is the most common route of exposure; other routes are ingestion, skin contact, and injection.

Organic mercury is usually found in fish and other aquatic organisms, but also occurs in produce, livestock, processed grains, and dairy products. Most commonly, humans are exposed to mercury by inhaling fumes from dental fillings or eating fish with high mercury concentrations (to name a few in the *"danger zone"* with highest concentrations: king mackerel, shark, swordfish, tilefish; fish in the *"caution zone"* with middle concentrations: bass, bluefish, halibut, lobster, orange roughy, snapper, tuna; fish in the *"your best bet zone"* with lowest concentrations: anchovies, cod, carp, clams, haddock, oyster, salmon, scallops, tilapia, whitefish). Symptoms of mercury exposure include abdominal cramps, vomiting, diarrhea, constipation, bloating, flatulence, loss of appetite, obesity, and hemorrhage.

HOW TO ELIMINATE TOXINS FROM HEAVY METALS

o Get tested (hair, saliva, or blood) by a chiropractor or natural health care practitioner.

o Have your mercury amalgams removed.

o Use ion foot baths, which neutralize heavy metal toxins.

o Reduce your aluminum exposure.

o Eat only safe fish.

o Don't get vaccinations or flue shots (both are toxic and contaminated).

o Do an Oxygen Colon Cleanse, then three back-to-back, liver and gallbladder cleanses. (See Resources.)

CADMIUM is an extremely toxic heavy metal. People are exposed by smoking or eating food products contaminated by industrial operations. Serious health problems can result, including colorectal cancer. Avoid common cadmium-containing food sources such as shelled seeds, organ meats, cabbage, and potato chips.

ALUMINUM (not a true heavy metal) is *incredibly toxic*, even in small amounts, and is used in many products. It can be absorbed through the intestinal tract or the lungs, depending on the route of exposure.

Drinking a can of soda dumps aluminum toxins into the gastrointestinal tract; the aluminum is slowly absorbed and can wind up in other tissues in the body. Ingestion of foods heated in aluminum cookware is suspected of contributing to colon inflammation; replace it with natural pots and pans (silicone bakeware and utensils, cast iron, stainless steel, or lead-glaze-free terra cotta). Use natural antiperspirants and deodorants that contain no aluminum.

Eliminating Intestinal Toxins from Radiation

Even though you can't see, smell, taste, or feel radiation, it's a real danger. Advanced research is being conducted on our everyday exposure to radiation, and much of it is bad news. Electromagnetic radiation (often called just "radiation") is energy emitted in the form of rays, or waves. Power lines, cell phones, computers, transformers, fluorescent lights, clock radios, and even hair dryers are only a few of the modern devices that emit dangerous electromagnetic waves. All your interactions with such devices add up, increasing your risk of developing several cancers, including colon cancer; they also overstress the colon and disrupt digestive processes, leading to abdominal pain, constipation, or diarrhea.

When electromagnetic radiation comes into contact with matter, it causes ionization, the loss of electrons in the atoms or molecules of matter. This process affects DNA and can result in cellular damage, chromosomal mutation, or even cell death. If losing electrons negatively affects a cell, then it affects tissue, which will affect organs. The body needs to *gain* electrons to stay healthy. You gain them by walking in the woods or along the beach, breathing pure oxygen, and eating live fruits and vegetables, among other ways.

Many common household electronics radiate harmful levels of electromechanical frequencies (EMFs). The combined effect of using various devices can damage the ultrasensitive colon, disrupt digestion, create colon toxicity, and make the colon susceptible to tumors. Even cell phone use can result in serious health complications, including cancer; never wear a mobile phone on a waist clip or in your pocket. Nonelectronic items (like wire bras, or metal bed frames) can also increase the amount of radiation emitted from an electronic source. Jobs associated with excessive radiation exposure include welders, electricians, machinists, TV repairers, phone cable splicers, and workers using fluorescent lights.

HOW TO REDUCE TOXINS FROM RADIATION

○ Use a cell phone only when necessary, and keep calls short. Use an EMF protection device on your cell phone, to reduce over 90% of the radiation it emits. On a regular phone, use the speakerphone.

○ Turn off electronics such as TVs and computers when not in use. Sit as far away from appliances as possible, and limit the amount of time you're using them.

○ Attach an EMF protection device to your computer to reduce over 90% of radiation emitted. Never set a laptop on your lap.

○ Replace all fluorescent lighting and standard light bulbs with full-spectrum lighting or LED lights.

○ Ladies, do not wear wire bras.

○ Avoid using microwaves and electric kettles. Reduce use of electric shavers.

Eliminating Intestinal Toxins from Parasites

Although it sustains life, the colon also provides a welcoming environment for dangerous invaders such as bacteria, viruses, yeasts, and worms. These organisms can enter the human body through air, soil, food, and water. *Everyone* is affected by parasites at some point. Luckily, you can take steps to rid your body of these invaders, and you'll enjoy increased energy levels and better well-being.

Parasites are a large and very real problem throughout the world, even in developed countries. If you think you can't get a parasite, think again. Experts estimate that *9 in 10 people have higher than normal levels of parasites in their bodies*. You might associate "parasite" with worms, but the two are not always the same. By definition, parasites are organisms that live on or inside another organism, called a "host," without making a useful return for its dependence. These invaders can range from microscopic amoebas, bacteria, fungi, and viruses to long, intestinal worms. They compete with you for nutrients and excrete toxic wastes that can threaten your health. They can further damage your body as they migrate and encyst themselves in protective shells in search of food and better shelter.

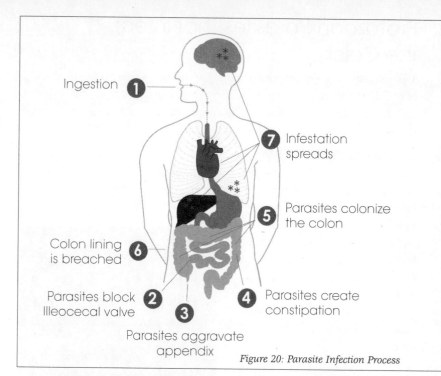

Figure 20: Parasite Infection Process

SOME HEALTH CONDITIONS CAUSED BY PARASITES

- Constipation
- Diarrhea
- Abdominal pain
- Flatulence
- Irritable bowel syndrome
- Dermatitis
- Allergies
- Sleeping problems
- Joint and muscle pain
- Nervousness
- Anemia
- Teeth grinding
- Fatigue
- Unexplained weight loss
- Colon cancer
- A chronically weakened immune system

Protozoan Parasites That Infect the Colon

The parasites briefly described below can be dangerous to the health of the intestinal tract. They feed off the vital nutrients from the body and destroy the permeability of the colon, and they emit harmful toxins inside you when they "go to the bathroom."

GIARDIA LAMBLIA

Protective cysts form around the parasite and their eggs, interfering with the host's fat digestion and preventing the absorption of important fat-soluble nutrients. Second only to bacterial invasion, giardiasis is the most common cause of diarrhea in North America. Symptoms of infection include severe diarrhea, bloating, flatulence (gas), abdominal cramping, weight loss, greasy stools, and dehydration. Day care centers are highly susceptible.

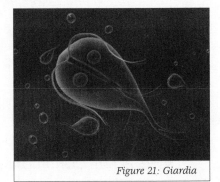

Figure 21: Giardia

TOXOPLASMA

People can become infected by eating contaminated meat and through contact with infected cat feces. A pregnant woman infected with toxoplasmosis can pass the disease to her fetus, who may develop serious conditions. Sixty million people in the United States are hosts to the toxoplasma parasite. Healthy individuals with uncompromised immune systems often show no symptoms, yet those with weakened immune systems can suffer from damage to the eyes, liver, lungs, heart, or brain.

CYCLOSPORA CAYETANENSIS

Symptoms of this parasite include diarrhea, loss of appetite, weight loss, bloating, gas, stomach pain, nausea, vomiting, muscle aches, fever, and fatigue. Once inside the body, cyclospora parasites invade the intestinal tract, where they mature and multiply at an alarming rate.

TAPEWORM

Tapeworms can survive in the body for 10 years and can grow to 30 feet in length. Consuming undercooked infected meat (such as pork, beef, or fish) can pass the parasite on to a human. Symptoms of infection include diarrhea, abdominal cramping, nausea, and appetite changes.

Tapeworms in infected sushi and other raw fish can lay up to a million eggs a day. Regular colon cleansing can flush out most tapeworms and their eggs.

ROUNDWORM FAMILY

Roundworms exist in over 20,000 observed species, 75 percent of which are parasitic and could affect you. More than *one billion people* are infected with roundworms, the most common intestinal parasite on the planet.

HOOKWORMS can penetrate the human skin, which allows them to enter the body through the feet of people who walk barefoot on soil contaminated by fecal matter (such as at a beach or on an animal farm). Symptoms of infection are stomach pain, loss of appetite, nausea, constipation, diarrhea, blood in the stool, gas, itchy skin, fever, and fatigue.

PINWORMS are small, white, intestinal parasites whose eggs travel to the small intestine to hatch and live for months.

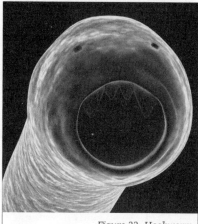

Figure 22: Hookworm

Symptoms are anal itchiness, insomnia, and appetite disruption caused by the laying of eggs around the anus, *not* by the worms themselves. Transmission can occur through contaminated clothing, toilets, bed linens, or other surfaces housing the parasites. Some 40 million Americans get them.

TRICHINELLA worms cause the disease trichinosis, which leads to many physical ailments such as muscle soreness, fever, diarrhea, nausea, vomiting, edema of the lips and face, difficulty breathing or speaking, enlarged lymph glands, fatigue, and dehydration. Eating raw or undercooked pork is usually the cause of trichinella infection in humans.

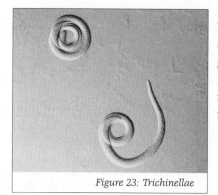

Figure 23: Trichinellae

A Fungus That Can Affect the Colon

Candida albicans is a yeast fungus that naturally inhabits the body; 90 percent of this fungus in the human body lives in the mouth and intestinal tract. Under the wrong conditions, *Candida* can grow out of control and have devastating effects on several areas of the body. Symptoms are abdominal pain, indigestion and bloating, constipation, food allergies, inability to think clearly, fatigue, itchy eyes, sinus drainage, muscle and joint pain, toenail and fingernail fungus, skin rashes, headaches, urinary tract infections, weight change, decreased sex drive, hair loss, menstrual irregularities, and depression.

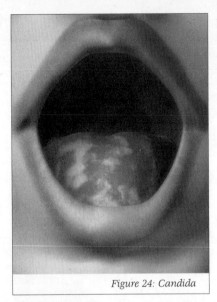

Figure 24: Candida

Having a small amount of *Candida* in your system is not a problem, for it behaves like a natural antibiotic and helps control the growth of harmful bacteria in the body. But 80 percent of people have serious *Candida* infections.

Bacteria and Viruses That Are Toxic to the Colon

The colon naturally accommodates billions of bacteria that help digest starches and convert them into energy and those fatty acids that are necessary in a healthy, cancer-free colon. These "good" bacteria also absorb nutrients and help prevent the growth of "bad" bacteria. But certain bad bacteria, such as *E. coli* and *Clostridia*, can putrefy meat inside the large intestine, turning it into cancer-causing agents.

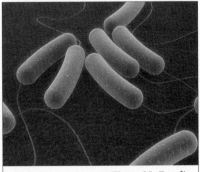

Figure 25: E. coli

Some strains of *E. coli* are benign, but others can cause serious and sometimes fatal health problems, such as kidney failure and hemolytic-uremic syndrome in children. Undercooked ground beef, contaminated water, and contaminated raw milk are sources of infection. Symptoms include bloody diarrhea, abdominal cramps, nausea, and vomiting.

Salmonella can cause typhoid fever and gastroenteritis. Salmonellosis is transmitted through direct contact with contaminated food, water, and fecal matter and can be picked up in a variety of places. Symptoms include headache, diarrhea, abdominal pain, fever, nausea, and vomiting; death can occur. The bacterium can be present in raw

---

HOW TO ELIMINATE TOXINS FROM PARASITES

○ Wash or peel fruits and vegetables. Scrape off any waxy coatings and cut out nicked areas. Buy organic.

○ Cook meats and fish to the appropriate temperature. (Read labels, and use a meat thermometer.) Check especially fish for worms underneath the skin. Wash hands carefully after handling raw meats and fish, and keep work surfaces and utensils clean (to avoid cross-contamination).

○ Know your water source. Drink only pure water from a treated, filtered source, or purified or distilled water that you've supplemented with organic apple cider vinegar.

○ Wash hands often. Warm water and natural tea tree soap can help remove any parasites. Clean under fingernails. Wash hands *before* eating and cooking and *after* handling raw foods, using the toilet, caring for pets, or changing a diaper.

○ Keep living area clean. Parasites can thrive in dust, soil particles, and fecal matter from dust mites and cockroaches. Remove dust frequently with a dampened sponge or a HEPA vacuum cleaner. Wash sheets and other bedding in hot water every few days. Get an indoor air filter.

○ Wear shoes when outdoors. Parasites can enter the body through the soles of the feet, so keep feet covered at a beach or playground that may harbor contaminated animal waste.

○ Wear gloves when gardening, and wash hands when finished (parasites may be in the soil).

○ Be careful about where you choose to swim. Never swallow water while swimming, whether in a river, lake, or swimming pool. Chlorine does *not* kill most parasites. Avoid swimming if you have any open cuts or sores.

○ Supplement with a good probiotic to help balance the gut flora.

○ Do a thorough parasite cleanse 2 times a year. The normal life cycle of most parasites is six weeks, so it will take that long to do a complete cleanse.

○ Eat a balanced diet to regulate your colon pH.

○ Eliminate or reduce *all* the toxins discussed in this book.

○ Cleanse your colon regularly. Use natural remedies when possible. (See Resources section.)

meats, poultry, and eggs; unpasteurized dairy products; fish, shrimp, and frog legs; coconut; sauces and salad dressings; chocolate; and peanut butter.

How Do I Get Rid of All These Harmful Organisms?

Your body is subjected to a massive amount of toxins from intestinal invaders each and every day. Parasites can potentially contribute more toxins to your colon than any other source (including food, water, and air). They live, breed, feed, and excrete toxic waste inside your body 24 hours a day.

A strong, healthy immune system can help to repel many organisms that invade the human body. Your best defense is to take measures to keep harmful organisms away from your body in the first place.

Afterword

After everything I have shared with you, I'd like to express my hope that you will use this book as a guide and practice the toxin-reducing techniques it contains. Preventing disease and regaining your health starts in the colon. *Please don't wait until it is too late.* Pass this information on to your friends, family, colleagues, and loved ones. They will surely appreciate your concern for their health and happiness.

While this is a book focusing on colon cleansing, I have one final thought: I can tell you from experience that to restore health, you must do a full liver, gallbladder, intestinal, parasite, and heavy metal cleanse.

This book has shared with you the "Secret to Health." The secret for regaining your health and preventing disease from ravaging the body can be reduced to only seven words:

Intestinal / Liver / Gallbladder / Parasite / Heavy Metal: *Cleansing*

The trick to make this secret work for you is that you must continue cleansing until your health is restored. This means you may have to perform as many as 10 full cleanses, back to back. But now, as a result of developments that I have told you about in the book, you can speed the process up by using high-quality supplements that assist in the vital process of regenerating cells.

Bear in mind these final words—indeed, they are words to *live* by:

> *Every physician should realize that the intestinal toxaemias are the most important primary and contributing causes of many disorders and diseases of the human body.*

You will be astonished to learn that this statement was written in 1933, by Dr. Anthony Bassler, a world-renowned gastroenterologist who, over the course of 25 years, studied more than 5,000 cases of disease. I believe these words remain true today, even in a new millennium.

Take these words to heart, re-read this book often and practice its wisdom, and please accept my best wishes for a long and healthy life.

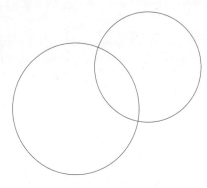

Glossary

Biliary system: The gallbladder and the ducts that carry bile and other digestive enzymes from the liver, gallbladder, and pancreas to the small intestine.

Bioengineering: An alteration produced by modifying the genetic structure of a biological process or organism.

Biorhythms: Biological cycles that follow a rhythm or pattern.

Body pH: Refers to the measurement of the body's acidity or alkalinity.

Carcinogen: A foreign substance that causes cancer.

Degenerative disease: A state of disease in which the affected tissues progressively deteriorate over time.

Detoxify: To cleanse the body of accumulated toxins.

Endocrine system: The system of glands that function to regulate bodily processes. These glands include the hypothalamus, pineal, pituitary, thyroid, parathyroid, and adrenal glands.

Enzymes: Special proteins produced by living organisms that function as biochemical catalysts.

Epidemiological: The branch of medicine that addresses disease.

Essential fatty acids: Fats required by the body that humans can get only from food.

Gluten and celiac disease: This disease (also called CD) is unique in that a specific food component, gluten, has been identified as the trigger. Gluten is the common name for the offending proteins in specific cereal grains that are harmful to persons with celiac disease.

Hemorrhoids: Painful, enlarged veins in the anal area that can generate enough discomfort to discourage regular bowel movements.

Impacted waste: The accumulation of hard compacted fecal matter that builds up from years of poor dietary and environmental choices. This matter adheres to the walls of the intestines and is not eliminated during regular bowel movements.

Lipase: A digestive enzyme that breaks down fats in the body.

Lutein: A pigment that helps protect against eye disease.

Niacin (nicotinic acid): Part of the vitamin B complex made from the oxidation of nicotine.

Noxious: Having qualities that are harmful to living creatures.

Refined: Food that has undergone chemical or mechanical manipulation before being consumed.

Serotonin: A chemical hormone that carries messages from one part of the body to another and helps regulate emotions, body temperature, sexuality, and appetite, as well as bowel movements.

Synergistic: The relationship between compounds or systems in which their combined effect is greater than that of the sum of its parts.

Synthesize: To artificially create something whole by combining individual elements.

Synthetic B vitamins: Type of B vitamins that are produced from coal tar (a nonliving substance potentially toxic to the body).

Toxic colon: Simply put, a colon that has been damaged by toxic substances that harm the lining, causing injury or illness.

Type II diabetes: Condition resulting from insufficient amounts of insulin and leading to excessive glucose (sugar) levels.

Resources

The following resources are listed in alphabetical order, not chapter order. Feel free to contact the author's Global Healing Center—*www.ghchealth.com/contact;* or call (800) 476-0016—if you need help finding high-quality supplements, products, and healthful alternatives for common foods and materials.

ABDOMINAL MASSAGE

Colon Cleansing & Constipation Resource Center, *www.colon-cleanse-constipation.com/colon-massage.html;* (800) 476-0016

Health-Choices Holistic Massage Therapy School; (908) 359-3995

Maya Abdominal Massage, www.arvigomassage.com; (603) 588-2571

AIR CONDITIONERS (AND FILTERS)

Change your air conditioner filters every month if you have pets, every other month if you don't. Learn more by visiting *www.onlineallergyrelief.com.* Get regular adjustments from a chiropractor to keep the nerve pathways to the bowels functioning properly and relieve stress.

AIR QUALITY

Use a quality air purification system that incorporates UV, negative ions, and HEPA filter technology. Surround Air and Way Healthier Home are excellent brands.

Surround Air, *www.surroundair.com;* (888) 812-1516

Mercola, *www.mercola.com/forms/air_purifiers.htm;* (877) 985-2695

ALLERGIES (AND RELIEF OF)

NAET Allergy Elimination Technique, *www.naet.com*; (714) 523-8900

ALOE VERA JUICE

R PUR Aloe International, *www.rpuraloe.com*; (800) 888-2563

Global Healing Center, *www.ghchealth.com/aloe_vera_juice.php*; (800) 476-0016

APPLE CIDER VINEGAR

Solana Gold Organics, *www.solanagold.com*

Bragg Live Food Products, *www.bragg.com*; (800) 446-1990

Spectrum Organic Products, *www.spectrumorganics.com*

BEDDING AND PILLOWS

Green Culture, www.greenculture.com; (877) 204-7336

EcoBedroom, www.ecobedroom.com; (626) 969-3707

BREAD

Alive and Well, *www.yahwehsaliveandwell.com*; (386) 437-0020

Diamond Organics, *www.diamonrdorganics.com*; (888) 674-2642

Heartland Mill, *www.heartlandmill.com*; (800) 232-8533

CARPET (AND CLEANING OF)

Use nontoxic hardwood flooring or nontoxic wool carpeting. If you cannot afford to replace all your carpet, use all-natural carpet cleaning supplies. You can purchase these at your local health food stores or from:

Naturell Carpet and Upholstery Cleaning, *www.bio-techan.com/carpet.htm*; (800) 468-3971

Nirvana Safe Haven, www.nontoxic.com; (800) 968-9355

These Vacuums Suck; www.thesevacuumssuck.com; (800) 248-1987

Vacuum Center, www.thevacuumcenter.com; (877) 224-9998

CELLULAR DEVICES (AND RADIATION FROM)

Everyone should have an EMF protection device on his or her cell phone.

Exradia, www.exradia.com

Global Healing Center, www.ghchealth.com/cell-phone-emf.php

Mercola, www.mercola.com/forms/ferrite_beads.htm

CLEANSERS AND DEGREASERS

Learn more about organic alternatives to toxic, commercial cleansers at:

Citrisolve, *www.citrisolve.com*; (800) 556-6785

Greenearth Cleaning, *www.greenearthcleaning.com*; (816) 926-0895

Heather's Naturals, *www.heathersnaturals.com*; (877) 527-6601

Seventh Generation, *www.seventhgeneration.com*; (800) 456-1191

COFFEE

Substitute store-bought coffee with natural grain coffee—a ground mixture of grains, nuts, and dried fruit, and providing only natural flavors—or herbal blends such as:

Teeccino, *www.teeccino.com*; (800) 498-3434

Bambu, *www.mehndiskinart.com/Bambu_Coffee_Substitute.htm*; (250) 664-6483

Pero, *www.internaturalfoods.com/Pero/Pero.html*; (973) 338-1499

Caffe Roma, *www.cafferoma.com*; (415) 296-7662

COLON (AND THE STRUCTURE AND FUNCTION OF)

A.D.A.M. Healthcare Center, *adam.about.com/encyclopedia/Structure-of-the-colon.htm*

Colon Cleansing and Constipation Resource Center, *www.colon-cleanse-constipation.com*; (800) 476-0016

COLON (AND TOXICITY AND DISEASES OF)

Colon Cleansing & Constipation Resource Center, *www.colon-cleanse-constipation.com*; (800) 476-0016

COLON CLEANSING (AND CLEANSERS)

Learn more about colon cleansing supplements in general by visiting these product review and informational sites:

Colon Cleansing & Constipation Resource Center, *www.colon-cleanse-constipation.com/best-colon-cleanse.html*; (800) 476-0016

Colon Cleansing Report Card, *www.coloncleansingreportcard.com*

Colon Cleansing Review, *coloncleansingreview.com/index.html*

Natural Healing Today, *www.naturalhealingtoday.com/colon_cleanse_product_reviews.html*

Relieving Constipation Naturally, *relievingconstipationnaturally.com/colon-cleanser.html*

COLONIC HYDROTHERAPY

International Association for Colon Hydrotherapy, *www.i-act.org*; (210) 366-2888

International School for Colon Hydrotherapy; (800) 717-7432

COOKING OIL

Replace with organic sources of virgin coconut oil, olive oil, grapeseed oil, almond oil, and peanut oil, available at:

Mercola, *www.mercola.com/forms/coconut_oil.htm*; (877) 985-2695

Organic Oil, *organicoil.com/default.aspx*; (888) 421-6546

Spectrum Organics, *www.spectrumorganics.com/?id=6*

Wilderness Family Naturals, *www.wildernessfamilynaturals.com*; (866) 936-6457

COOKWARE

Avoid aluminum, Teflon-coated, copper, and stainless steel (inferior grades contain Nickel to reduce costs) cookware. I recommend glass, terracotta (without lead glaze), titanium, silicone, or cast iron cookware.

Castiron Cookware, *www.castironcookware.com*

Le Creuset, *www.lecreuset.com/usa/home.php*; (877) 273-8738

DUST MITES

Check your bedding for dust mites in 10 minutes using the Mite-T-Fast home test kit; *www.avehobiosciences.com/products.shtml;* (866) 590-0972.

EXERCISE

I recommend the following exercises and physical activities for helping to reduce stress and improve overall health:

Balanced Body (Pilates). *www.pilates.com;* (800) 745-2837

Qigong (meditative exercise), National Qigong Association (NQA), *www.nqa.org;* (888) 815-1893

Rebounding (jumping on mini-trampolines)

Cellercise Rebounding, *www.cellercise.com;* (800) 856-4863

Jumpsport, *www.jumpsport.com;* (888) 567-5867

Jump 4 Health, *www.jump4health.com;* (888) 815-3332

Walking Healthy, *www.walkinghealthy.com*

Yoga Finder, *www.yogafinder.com;* (858) 213-7924

International Association of Yoga Therapists, *www.iayt.org;* (928) 541-0004

FOOD (GENERAL)

Shop at your local farmers markets. All chain-store or national supermarkets stock foods shipped in from distant suppliers. This means the fruit and vegetables are picked before they have ripened and matured to their full nutrient potential. Local farmers' markets, however, pick the food fresh and ripened and deliver it fresh every day or two.

FOOD (STORAGE)

Store food in nontoxic containers. Use glass Pyrex containers with silicone lids to reduce contamination from common plastic containers and plastic wraps; *www.pyrexware.com,*

GALLBLADDER CLEANSING

Global Healing Center, *www.ghchealth.com/cleansing*

GENETICALLY MODIFIED FOODS

For an extensive list of foods and brands containing GMOs, visit *www.truefoodnow.org;* (415) 826-2770

HEAVY METALS (AND CLEANSING OF FROM THE BODY)

Medicardium, *www.medicardium.com;* (888) 456-4268

BioRay, *www.bioray2000.com/home.cfm;* (888) 635-9582

Newstarget, *www.newstarget.com/015232.html*

LAXATIVES

Oxy-Powder, *www.oxypowder.com/articles/warning-herbal-cleanser.html;* (800) 476-0016

Colon Cleansing & Constipation Resource Center, *www.colon-cleanse-constipation.com/laxatives.html;* (800) 476-0016

LIVER CLEANSING

Global Healing Center, *www.ghchealth.com/cleansing*

MEAT

Buy organic, range-fed, hormone-and antibiotic-free meat.

Applegate Farms, www.applegatefarms.com; (866) 587-5858

Blackwing Quality Meats, www.blackwing.com; (800) 326-7874

The Meatrix, *www.themeatrix.com;* (212) 991-1930

NorthStar Bison, *www.northstarbison.com;* (888) 295-6332

MEDICINE (GENERAL)
To learn more about natural health care and avoiding toxins from drugs, visit American College for Advancement in Medicine, *www.acam.org;* (800) 532-3688

MICROWAVES
Always grill, steam, broil, or bake your food in the oven. Replace your microwave with an air-convection oven; *www.comrpactappliance.com;* (800) 297-6076.

MILK (AND DAIRY PRODUCTS)
Buy organic, range-fed, hormone- and antibiotic-free dairy products. Replace cow's milk with hemp milk, rice milk, fermented soymilk, almond milk, or raw goat's milk.

Organic Pastures Dairy Company, *www.organicpastures.com;* (877) 729-6455

Organic Valley Farmers' Raw Cheese, www.organicvalley.coop; (888) 444-6455

Why Real Milk?, *www.realmilk.com;* (202) 363-4394

For an easy recipe for hemp milk, visit *nutiva.com/nutrition/recipes/milk.php;* (800) 993-4367

MOLD AND MILDEW
If you live in a high-humidity area, dehumidify the house at least twice a week. In Australia, tea tree oil is commonly used in ventilation systems to control bacteria and mold growth, available at *www.mountainroseherbs.com/aroma/q-z.html;* (800) 879-3337.

Other essential oils can be purchased at *www.libertynatural.com;* (800) 289-8427.

Have your home tested for mold spores, particularly if you live in a humid area. Test kits are available at *www.HomeMoldTestKit.com;* (877) 665-3373.

Use a high-quality air purification system that includes UV, negative ions, and HEPA filter technology. The Germicidal UV lamp is the most effective air purification method available for destroying microorganisms like viruses, bacteria, and fungi such as mold.

NATURAL PESTICIDES
Beyond Pesticides, *www.beyondpesticides.org;* (202) 543-5450

Organic Pesticides, *www.organicpesticides.com;* (805) 927-7400

OXYGEN COLON CLEANSER
Dreddy Clinic, *www.dreddyclinic.com/products/oxygen-colon-cleansers.htm*

Oxy-Powder®, *www.oxypowder.com;* (800) 476-0016

Colon Cleansing & Constipation Resource Center, *www.colon-cleanse-constipation.com/oxygen-colon-cleansers.html;* (800) 476-0016

PARASITES (AND THE REDUCTION OF VIA THOROUGH HAND WASHING)
Wash your hands frequently throughout the day. Warm water and natural tea tree soap can help remove any microscopic parasites with which you have come into contact. Clean in and beneath fingernails as well. Organic soaps are available at:

Herbaria, *www.herbariasoap.com*

Global Healing Center, *www.ghchealth.com/organic-skin-care*

Soap For Goodness Sake, *www.soapforgoodnesssake.com*

PARASITES (AND THE REMOVAL OF WITH HEALTH SUPPLEMENTS)

Help create an environment within your body that is inhospitable for potential invaders. Learn more about cleansing supplements and protocols at:

Global Healing Center, *www.ghchealth.com/paratrex.php;* (800) 476-0016

www.colon-cleanse-constipation.com/liver-flush-gallbladder-flush.html

PESTICIDE-CONTAINING FOODS

For a list of pesticide-containing foods, *visit www.ewg.org;* (510) 444-0973.

PET DANDER

Vacuum and wash all bedding frequently using an all-natural laundry detergent and a vacuum with a HEPA filter. Learn about a natural alternative to chemical detergent at *www.maggiespureland.com/product.html;* (888) 762-7688.

Use an excellent air purification system that includes UV, negative ion, and HEPA filtration.

PROBIOTICS

Latero-Flora, *www.ghchealth.com/probiotic-bacterium-supplement.php;* (800) 476-0016

RADIATION (AND DETECTION OF)

Use a detector to check the levels of radiation in your home and workplace.

Radalert 100, *www.geigercounters.com/Radalert.htm*

SALT

Replace table salt with natural Himalayan Salt or Celtic Sea Salt.

www.mercola.com/forms/salt.htm; (877) 985-2695

www.celticseasalrt.com; (800) 867-7258

You can also use Braggs Liquid Aminos to flavor dishes you would normally salt, *www.bragg.com/products/liquidaminos.html;* (800) 446-1990.

SEAFOOD

Avoid questionable-source seafood (especially shellfish).

Rose Fisheries, *www.rosefisheries.com;* (877) 747-3107

Vital Choice Seafood, *www.vitalchoice.com;* (800) 608-4825

SOY

Use organic fermented sources such as natto (fermented soybeans), tempeh, tofu, miso, or tamari, available at:

www.edenfoods.com/store/product_info.php?products_id=107580; (888) 424-3336

www.soyboy.com/index.htm; (585) 235-8970

www.san-j.com/product_list.asp?id=1; (800) 446-5500

SQUATTING PLATFORM

Lillipad, lillipad.co.nz

Nature's Platform, *www.naturesplatform.com;* (828) 297-7561

SUGAR AND ARTIFICIAL SWEETENERS

Replace refined sugars and artificial sweeteners (saccharin, neotame, acesulfame potassium, aspartame, and sucralose) with organic agave nectar, xylitol, raw cane sugar, or locally grown unprocessed honey.

Agave Nectar, *www.madhavahoney.com;* (303) 823-5166

Brown Rice Syrup, *www.auntpattys.com;* (800) 456-7923

Organic Maple Syrup, *www.maplevalleysyrup.com;* (800) 760-1449

YS Organic Bee Farm, *www.ysorganic.com;* (800) 654-4593

SWIMMING POOLS AND FILTRATION

The ECOsmarte system uses copper ions and ozone to purify the water; *www.ecosmarte.com;* (800) 466-7946.

VOLATILE ORGANIC COMPOUNDS

Purchase nontoxic paints from alternative companies, available at:

www.ecosorganicpaints.com

www.greenplanetpaints.com; (520) 394-2571

www.realmilkpaint.com; (800) 339-9748

WATER (AND TESTING FOR ARSENIC)

PurTest Arsenic Test is a simple home-screening kit for this heavy metal; *purtest.com/ 2007%20kits.htm;* (704) 821-3200.

WATER (BATHING/SHOWERING)

Install shower and bath filters—remember, your skin absorbs toxins. I recommend the Wellness shower filter; *www.ghchealth.com/wellness-shower-filter.php;* (800) 476-0016.

WATER (GENERAL TESTING)

Test your water for contaminants with a home water test kit; *www.ghchealth.com/water-testing-kit.php;* (800) 476-0016.

WATER (PURIFICATION AND DRINKING)

The Wellness Carafe is a high-quality portable water purifier you can take with you anywhere to purify water; available at *www.ghchealth.com/wellness-water-carafe.php.*

Learn more about Wellness Water and other water purification methods by visiting *www.ghchealth.com/water-purification.*

Oxygen water is purified water with the additional benefit of providing oxygen to your system; *www.o2techno.com;* (201) 943-6900.

Additional Recommended Reading

Marcia Angell, M.D., *The Truth About Drug Companies: How They Deceive Us and What to Do About It* (Random House Trade Paperbacks, 2005)

E. Batmanghelidj, M.D., *Water Cures: Drugs Kill: How Water Cured Incurable Diseases*

Christopher Bryson, *Fluoride Deception* (Seven Stories Press, 2004)

Stephen Fried, *Bitter Pills: Inside the Hazardous World of Legal Drugs* (Bantam, 1998)

Daniel Haley, *Politics in Healing: The Suppression and Manipulation of American Medicine* (Potomac Valley Press, 2000)

Ralph W. Moss, Ph.D., *The Cancer Industry* (Paragon House, 1991)

Dr. James R. Walker, *Holocaust American Style*

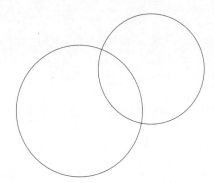

Index

Other Books from Ulysses Press

The Complete Master Cleanse: A Step-by-Step Guide to Maximizing the Benefits of The Lemonade Diet
Tom Woloshyn, $11.95
Fasting for days while drinking a lemonade-like blend of clear spring water, cayenne pepper and citrus juice has proven to be a safe, simple and yet powerful way to cleanse the body of toxins. This book goes beyond basic information on how to do the cleanse by guiding readers step by step through the entire cleansing process.

Irritable Bowel Syndrome: A Natural Approach
Third Edition, Rosemary Nicol foreword by William John Snape, $14.95
Clearly written with easy-to-understand explanations, this book presents natural solutions for living comfortably with this common ailment.

The Juice Fasting Bible: Discover the Power of an All-Juice Diet to Restore Good Health, Lose Weight and Increase Vitality
Sandra Cabot, M.D., $12.95
Offering a series of quick and easy juice fasts, this book provides a reader-friendly approach to an increasingly popular, alternative health practice.

The Liver and Gallbladder Miracle Cleanse: An All-Natural, At-Home Flush to Purify and Rejuvenate Your Body
Andreas Moritz, $14.95
Illustrates how to recognize stone buildup and provides do-it-yourself instructions for painlessly flushing them out of the body.

The pH Balance Diet: Restore Your Acid-Alkaline Levels to Eliminate Toxins and Lose Weight
Bharti Vyas & Suzanne Le Quesne, $12.95
Tells how to pH-test one's body, correct imbalances and eliminate toxic overload by following a dietary way of life that works. An easy-to-follow section with over 40 recipes is included to help guide readers through the plan.

To order these books call 800-377-2542 or 510-601-8301, fax 510-601-8307, e-mail ulysses@ ulyssespress.com, or write to Ulysses Press, P.O. Box 3440, Berkeley, CA 94703. All retail orders are shipped free of charge. California residents must include sales tax. Allow two to three weeks for delivery.

About
the Author

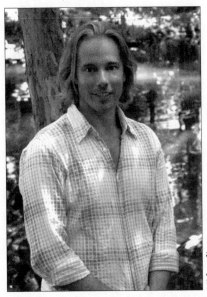

Nida Ali

Dr. Edward F. Group III holds doctorates of Chiropractic and Naturopathy and is a Diplomate of the American Clinical Board of Nutrition. He is also a Certified Clinical Nutritionist (CCN), a Certified Clinical Herbalist (CCH), and a Holistic Health Practitioner (HHP).

In 1998 Dr. Group founded Global Healing Center with the commitment to teach people how to heal themselves, prevent disease, and improve their general health and well-being. With him at the helm, the center has helped hundreds of thousands of people worldwide prevent or eliminate disease. Dr. Group also directs the product development team and assumes a hands-on approach in formulating advanced and effective organic and natural health supplements.

Although he no longer sees patients directly, Dr. Group now educates millions of people via information technology. He has written numerous books and articles on myriad natural health care topics, has studied alternative medicine for over 20 years, and wants to share his discoveries with the world. This book is the culmination of his lifelong goal to provide the ultimate guide for restoring or achieving optimal health.

A recognized international health care speaker, Dr. Group has spoken along with Deepak Chopra, M.D.; Stedman Graham; Julian Whitaker, M.D.; Larry Dossey, M.D.; Don Miguel Ruiz; Darma Singh Khalsa, M.D.; Joseph Mercola, D.O.; Garry Gordon, M.D.; Christine Northrup, M.D.; Burton Goldberg; and other experts.

Dr. Group continues his health research and personal leadership of Global Healing Center in Houston, Texas. He may be contacted at *www.ghchealth.com* or by phone at (800) 476-0016 or (713) 476-0016.